CALCIUM AND
PHOSPHORUS METABOLISM

TO JANET

Calcium and Phosphorus Metabolism

JAMES T. IRVING

Department of Histology
Forsyth Dental Center
Boston, Massachusetts

With Chapters by
FELIX BRONNER

University of Connecticut Health Center
Storrs, Connecticut

GIDEON A. RODAN

University of Connecticut Health Center
Storrs, Connecticut

ACADEMIC PRESS New York and London 1973
A Subsidiary of Harcourt Brace Jovanovich, Publishers

ACADEMIC PRESS, INC.
111 Fifth Avenue, New York, New York 10003

United Kingdom Edition published by
ACADEMIC PRESS, INC. (LONDON) LTD.
24/28 Oval Road, London NW1

Library of Congress Cataloging in Publication Data

Irving, James Tutin, DATE
    Calcium and phosphorus metabolism.

    Bibliography: p.
    1.   Calcium metabolism.   2.   Phosphorus metabolism.
I.   Bronner, Felix.   II.   Rodan, Gideon A.
III.   Title.
[DNLM: 1.   Calcium—Metabolism.   2.   Phosphorus—
Metabolism.   QU 130 I72ca 1973]
QP535.C2177   612'.3924   72–88352
ISBN 0–12–374350–8

PRINTED IN THE UNITED STATES OF AMERICA

CONTENTS

PREFACE

Originally this monograph was planned as a second edition of "Calcium Metabolism," which was published in 1957, with information about phosphorus to be added. It was soon apparent that most of the work was out of date, so rapid have been the advances over the past fifteen years. As a result, the material comprising this book is almost completely new; only small parts of the original have been retained.

Only the metabolism of inorganic phosphorus is considered since a complete treatise on the physiology of this element, including the roles of the many organic phosphorus compounds which occur in the body, would be outside the scope of this monograph. Organic compounds are only incidentally mentioned.

I am most grateful to Drs. Bronner and Rodan for their respective chapters on "Kinetic and Cybernetic Analysis of Calcium Metabolism" and on "Cellular Functions of Calcium."

JAMES T. IRVING

————— *Chapter 1*

DIETARY SOURCES OF CALCIUM AND PHOSPHORUS

Of the solid elements, calcium and phosphorus are present in the body in the highest concentrations; this is surprising in view of their relative unavailability in nature. While calcium is widespread in rocks and soil, its insolubility probably accounts for the small amounts present in foods.

Calcium and phosphorus are present in bone and teeth in combination as members of the hydroxyapatite family, $Ca_{10}(PO_4)_6 \cdot (OH)_2$, and are also mainly present in the earth's crust in this form. This is fortunate, since our understanding of calcified tissues has benefited from work of geologists and crystallographers. By leaching of primary rocks on the earth's surface through geological time, a source has been provided for biological calcium phosphate formation. Posner (1969) has given interesting schemes of the marine and land calcium phosphate cycles.

Katchman (1961) has reviewed the occurrence of phosphorus in nature. It is present in water as orthophosphate, but in the soil it is very insoluble, in the form of apatite. However, enough CO_2 is present in water, in equilibrium with the CO_2 of the air, to make a small amount of phosphate soluble, and this phosphate can be used by plants and microorganisms that are present in the soil or the sea. They transform it into organic and inorganic compounds, and animals and man rely on this supply for dietary phosphorus either directly or through some other animal source. So vital is phosphorus for animals that in areas where phosphorus lack is endemic, the grazing animals take to eating soil and have other depraved appetites (Theiler and Green, 1931–1932).

The calcium and phosphorus contents of common foodstuffs have now been widely determined and many tables exist giving this information. The best sources of calcium and phosphorus in human diets is milk or milk products, with the exception of butter. In the reference book "Metabolism," published by the Federation of American Societies for Experimental Biology (Altman and Dittmer, 1968), cow's milk is reported to contain 0.12 g calcium and 0.10 g phosphorus/100 ml. In contrast, human milk contains only 0.032 and 0.015 g/100 ml, respectively, of the two elements. The composition of skim cow's milk is, as far as calcium and phosphorus are concerned, virtually the same as that of whole milk, the phosphorus being somewhat reduced. Human colostrum contains almost the same amount of calcium and phosphorus as human milk. Hard American cheese is an excellent source of both elements, containing 697 and 771 mg/100 g, respectively. Cottage creamed cheese has only about one seventh of that present in hard cheese.

Friend (1967) has made an intensive analysis of calcium intakes and milk consumption in this country. The dietary calcium content increased from 0.98 g/person/day in 1909–1913 to about 1 g in the 1940's, milk and milk products being the largest contributors of calcium. In the early 1900's they furnished about two thirds, and now provide three quarters of the intake. Calcium from fluid whole milk and evaporated milk has declined since the 1940's, but the intake of calcium supplied by such items are nonfat dry milk, ice cream and other frozen desserts, and cheese have increased considerably. Twardock et al. (1960), investigating goat's milk, found that 70–80% of the calcium was bound to caseinate, and about 80% of the rest was ultrafiltrable. Fairney and Weir (1970) reported that high calcium diets could increase the calcium of the milk of rats to a limited extent.

Most other items of the diet are poor suppliers of calcium, but often are rich in phosphorus. Thus meat containing only 13 mg calcium/

100 g could contain up to 200 mg phosphorus. Eggs are a good source of phosphorus (205 mg/100 g) and a fair source of calcium (54 mg/100 g). Green leafy vegetables are not in general a good source of calcium, the only item containing sizable amounts being turnip greens (246 mg/100 g raw, and 184 mg after boiling and draining), raw common cabbage containing 49 mg calcium and 29 mg phosphorus/100 g, and boiled drained spinach 93 mg calcium and 38 mg phosphorus. These figures are typical of several green leafy vegetables containing so little calcium and phosphorus as to make a meager contribution to the daily requirement. In addition, Krehl and Winters (1950) showed that boiling green vegetables could result in a loss of up to 25% of the contained calcium.

Certain nuts (e.g., almonds and hazel nuts) contain relatively high amounts of calcium and phosphorus, and cereal grains also contain much phosphorus, but probably a fraction of this is in the form of phytate.

It sometimes happens that unusual and unexpected sources of calcium are encountered. Thus, Baker and Mazess (1963), when investigating a Peruvian diet, found that it was the local custom to include a ground rock containing calcium and ashed grain stalks which were also rich in calcium. By these additions, the daily calcium could equal and sometimes exceed the recommended calcium allowance.

Several foods now have calcium added to them, the commonest being bread. In England, chalk is added to the flour to overcome the action of phytic acid, and in the United States dried milk and improvers are added, considerably increasing the calcium and phosphorus content (Altman and Dittmer, 1968).

Water as a Source of Calcium

Several studies have reported a negative correlation between the hardness of the drinking water and death from cardiovascular disease; as a result interest has been taken in the calcium content of water and the possible effect on sodium metabolism. A recent study by Hankin *et al.* (1970), undertaken in California, showed that soft water contributed about 3.5% of the total calcium intake, and hard water about 7%. The mean concentration of calcium was 5.0 mg/100 ml. A study in

England by Crawford *et al.* (1968) showed that the calcium content of the water they analyzed ranged from 9.0 to 11.4 mg/100 ml. Many years ago McCance and Widdowson (1943) concluded that only under conditions of low calcium intake would hard water make a significant contribution to the diet, and this is still the consensus.

Chapter 2

MECHANISM OF CALCIUM AND PHOSPHORUS ABSORPTION IN THE INTESTINE: THE ACTION OF VITAMIN D

Vitamin D

This vitamin, a sterol derivative, probably exists in several forms and is essential for adequate intestinal calcium absorption in most vertebrates. Originally it was supposed to be part of the growth fat-soluble vitamin found in cod liver oil, but McCollum _et al._ (1922) separated the antixerophthalmic and antirachitic factors and demonstrated that it was an independant entity. As described elsewhere, when the vitamin is absent from the body, the bone disease rickets occurs. It exists naturally as vitamin D_3 or cholecalciferol. This is formed in the animal from its precursor, 7-dehydrocholesterol, by ultraviolet irradiation of the skin, the precursor being in the sebaceous secretions. Ergosterol, when irradiated, is similarly transformed into a vitamin D, which is called D_2. These compounds are also called cholecalciferol and ergocalciferol, respectively, and the effect of irradiation is to open the second or B sterol ring, which confers vitamin activity on them. Vitamin D_2 was the first of these vitamins to be identified, but when it was found that cod liver oil was antirachitic in chicks whereas vitamin D_2 was not, the antirachitic fraction of cod liver oil was isolated and found to be a slightly different compound, now known as D_3.

An international unit has been established; the potency of both vitamin D_2 and D_3 is 40,000 IU/mg for mammals. In chicks vitamin D_3 has the same potency, but D_2 a potency of only 1000 IU/mg. An exception to this has been reported by Hunt *et al.* (1967), who found that while D_3 promoted calcium absorption in the new world monkey, *Cebus albifrons*, D_2 has no such action. Apart from certain fish liver oils, vitamin D is found in very few foods and only in small amounts. Thus mammalian liver contains only 1–4, egg yolk 1–5 IU/g, and milk 3–100 IU/liter. Most milk in the United States is fortified by dairy firms with vitamin D. Thus man largely relies on sunshine for his vitamin D; as a result the requirement is not accurately known. The National Research Council recommends an allowance for infants, children, and pregnant and lactating women of 400 IU/day, probably ample in infants, but requiring supplementation by sunshine in adults.

Calcium Absorption

The lumen of the small intestine is bounded with epithelial cells which under the light microscope have a striated border. Electron microscopy has revealed that this border is made up of microvilli, closely packed, 1–1.4 μm in length and 800 Å in diameter. On top of this is a surface coat, the brush border, consisting mostly of acid glycosaminoglycans, and about 0.1–0.5 μm wide. These structures probably play a significant role in calcium absorption.

This phenomenon has been much investigated over the last decade, and many of the investigations have used everted loops of small or large intestine in *in vitro* experiments. This method is not without its critics, especially as the ion studied has to penetrate not only the mucosa, but also the muscle layers and the serosa, to be estimated in the fluids inside the everted sac. Both Sallis and Holdsworth (1962) and Williams *et al.* (1962) have reported experiments indicating that the *in vivo* and *in vitro* behavior of intestinal loops of chicks and rats was not always identical. However, much useful information has been obtained from *in vitro* studies and thus this model must be regarded, when its limitations are realized, as a useful approach.

The modern pioneers of this method have been Schachter and his group. Schachter and Rosen (1959) and Schacter *et al.* (1960a) first described an active transport mechanism for calcium absorption against a concentration gradient. This process was relatively specific for calcium, not being found for other cations such as magnesium, strontium, barium, or potassium. This active transport was greater in preparations from young as compared to old rats, and in pregnant as compared to nonpregnant animals. In a later paper (1960b) they incubated intestinal slices with ^{45}Ca. The slices took up the labeled calcium in 1 hour to a concentration 5 times higher than that in the medium. This was inhibited by incubation in nitrogen or by the addition of dinitrophenol. Giving vitamin D before the intestine was removed greatly increased the calcium uptake. In 1961 Schachter *et al.* found that small doses of vitamin D_2 or D_3 given to vitamin-depleted rats restored the absorptive mechanism along the whole length of the small intestine, but especially in the duodenum. Oxidative metabolism was affected by vitamin D, which thus regulated an active mechanism controlling calcium transport rather than simple diffusion. Two processes were involved—uptake at the mucosal surface and efflux on the serosal side —and the vitamin was needed for both processes.

It should be stated here that vitamin D has no effect on calcium absorption if added to the medium of an *in vitro* preparation: It has to be administered to the intact animal before removal of the gut, and there is a lag period of some hours before its action can be observed, because it has to be transformed into active metabolites.

Dowdle *et al.* (1960) also reported that vitamin D pretreatment was necessary for active transport of calcium *in vitro*. This process was significantly increased by giving calciferol to vitamin D-depleted rats by stomach tube 1 hour before the experiment, vitamins D_2 and D_3 being equally effective. However, they gave an enormous dose of the vitamin (50,000 IU). Maintenance on a low calcium diet increased active transport. Active transport was an adaptive mechanism for adequate calcium absorption when more calcium was needed, or if the diet was low in calcium.

On the other hand, Harrison and Harrison (1960), also using everted intestinal loops, found that vitamin D given 72 hours previously to rachitic rats increased the rate of diffusion of calcium across the wall of the entire length of the small intestine. This process was not stopped by the inhibition of oxidative metabolism. Active transport occurred only in the proximal part of the intestine, and was dependent on oxidative metabolism.

The exact nature of this active transport has been much investigated. The question boils down to determining whether calcium entrance into the epithelial cell is involved, or its egress on the serosal side, or whether both are part of the mechanism, due regard being given to the fact that calcium may also leave the cell and go back into the intestinal lumen. Wasserman and Kallfelz (1962) used an *in vivo* preparation of the duodenum of rachitic chicks. Normally there were two fluxes: one, lumen to plasma; and the other plasma to lumen, the first being greater than the second. Vitamin D_3 increased both these fluxes, acting not on an unidirectional transport system, but on permeability changes of the mucosal cell. In a later paper, Wasserman *et al.* (1966), elaborating on this thesis, felt that vitamin D either modified membrane structure, or effected the synthesis of a calcium carrier. Rasmussen *et al.* (1963) studied calcium exchange in isolated intestinal villi of rats, and concluded there were three phenomena: an active uptake of calcium dependent on oxidative metabolism, a passive uptake dependent on the external calcium ion concentration, and a temperature-dependent calcium release. When incubated at 4° calcium was taken up, but on raising the temperature to 33°, calcium was released into the medium. Holdsworth (1965) developed a model in which the mucosal cell had two faces, luminal and serosal. Two pumps existed, driving calcium out of the cell into the lumen, or else out of the cell into the serosa, both operated by metabolic energy. Vitamin D inhibited the pump that returned calcium from the cell to the lumen. Walling and Rothman (1969) used a different technique with the intestine opened and mounted between two chambers. They found active transport in growing animals, but much less in adult rats. Inorganic phosphate was not necessary for the active transport to occur. A two-way flux existed and previous low calcium diets approximately doubled the flux from mucosa to serosa, but had no effect on the flux from serosa to mucosa, the low calcium effect being mediated by active transport. The mucosa–serosa transport could be saturated but the other flux could not be. This and the vitamin D dependence of the mucosa-to-serosa mechanism suggested the existence of a carrier-mediated calcium transport. Using a mucosal cell suspension, Hashim and Clark (1969) proposed that vitamin D was more concerned with the release from, rather than the uptake by, mucosal cells; this view was also held by Urban and Schedl (1970), using rat intestinal segments perfused *in situ*. They felt that the major effect of vitamin D was on a second or release step in the transport of calcium from the lumen to the bloodstream.

It will thus be seen that these various groups of workers developed quite different concepts of calcium absorption, and their views seem at present irreconcilable. These disagreements illustrate, in the judgment of the present writer, the disadvantages of *in vitro* techniques, and also of comparing different techniques.

On the question of the rate-limiting aspect of calcium absorption, there is more agreement. Walling and Rothman (1969) found that the transport mechanism, mucosa to serosa, could be saturated. On the basis of these findings, Patrick (1970), using slices of rat duodenum, proposed that the entry of calcium across the brush border was rate limiting in the absorption of calcium from lumen to plasma. He thought there was also an active transport across the basal border of the epithelial cells which was not rate limiting. The rate-limiting entry, which was energy dependent, allowed calcium translocation while preserving a low intracellular ionic calcium concentration (Papworth and Patrick, 1970).

Wensel *et al.* (1969) carried out an interesting study on normal humans. The intact small intestine was intubated and perfused. In the duodeno-jejunal area a calcium flux was apparent from lumen to blood even when the concentration in the lumen was below that in blood, the degree of the flux being positively correlated with the luminal calcium level. An ileal flux was also present; it was much lower and independent of the luminal calcium level. The flux from blood to lumen was low and also independent of the luminal calcium concentration. The flux lumen to blood was not altered by the administration of parathyroid hormone. The latter statement is of interest since Harrison and Harrison (1970) reported cyclic AMP to enhance calcium transport in rats, both *in vivo* and *in vitro*, but only if the animals had had adequate vitamin D.

Calcium-Binding Protein (CaBP)

An important advance was the discovery of calcium-binding proteins (CaBP) in the intestinal mucosa by Wasserman and his group. In 1966, Wasserman and Taylor reported the presence of such a protein in the mucosa of rachitic chicks given D_3 72 hours before sacrifice. Kallfelz *et al.* (1967), using rachitic rats, detected a CaBP 72 hours after giving vitamin D_2 or D_3, the mucosa of vitamin D-deficient rats having much less. Taylor and Wasserman (1967) isolated and partially purified the protein. It was found in all segments of the small intestine and also in the kidney of D_3-treated rachitic chicks (see also Sands and Kessler, 1971), but not in the colon, liver, or muscle; it was thus present in the soft tissues that were known physiological sites of vitamin D action. In the small intestine it was intimately associated with the transfer of calcium across the intestinal epithelium; Sands and Kessler thought that vitamin D might have as its first action a transcriptional effect on information transfer from the DNA system. Corradino and Wasserman (1968b), reported that the injection of actinomycin D, 2 hours before vitamin D administration to rachitic chicks, prevented the enhanced calcium absorption and the appearance of CaBP, thus confirming the possible transcriptional site of action of the vitamin.

The CaBP was also found in the intestinal mucosa of normal chicks, but in smaller amounts than that found after vitamin D treatment (Wasserman and Taylor, 1968). When rachitic but vitamin D_3-treated chicks were deprived of the vitamin, their calcium absorption and mucosal CaBP decreased in parallel. Chicks adapted to low calcium intakes had more CaBP than those not so adapted, young birds had more CaBP than older ones, and laying hens had more of the protein than nonlaying birds. Vitamin D_3 was more effective in promoting the formation of CaBP than was D_2.

Subsequent work by these authors has substantiated these findings. Four high affinity sites exist for calcium per molecule, and in addition numerous additional calcium-binding sites start to bind calcium when the concentration increases to 2×10^{-3} M (Bredderman, 1971). Immunofluorescent localization of the protein showed it to be in all segments of the small intestine, in the surface coat of the microvilli, and also in most of the PAS-positive and goblet cells. Lesser amounts were found in the colon. It was also seen in the kidney, but was absent from the blood plasma, liver, pancreas, and bone (Taylor and Wasserman, 1970). Corradino and Wasserman (1968a) also found a CaBP similar to that of the duodenum in the uterus of the laying hen. Recently Wasserman and Taylor (1971) reported that two New World monkeys, *Cebus* and the squirrel monkey, made a CaBP similar to that of other species, after vitamin D_3 treatment, the controls being on a rachitogenic diet.

Wasserman (1970) also proposed a mechanism for the release of calcium from CaBP. Lysolecithin caused a considerable reduction in the calcium-binding power of CaBP, and a phospholipase A has been found in the brush border of the intestine which could make lysolecithin available. Corradino and Wasserman (1970b) suggested an explanation of strontium rickets, since they found that this element inhibited the formation of CaBP.

Other workers have confirmed these results in whole or in part. Adams and Norman (1970) and Adams *et al.* (1970) have postulated that a carrier, present at the brush border, is altered in some way by vitamin D to effect a more efficient entry of calcium into the cell. Vitamin D caused a resynthesis of protein in the brush border membrane or a reorganization of the microvilli. Hamilton and Holdsworth (1970) considered that the CaBP caused the release of calcium from the mitochondria of intestinal mucosal cells. Extracts of intestine of vitamin D-deficient chicks did not cause this, since they contained no CaBP. Walling and Rothman (1970) reported that dietary calcium restriction caused an increased affinity for calcium in the carrier, rather than an increase in the capacity of the transport process. MacGregor *et al.* (1970), using rachitic chicks, found that vitamin D in small doses increased the incorporation of tritiated leucine into CaBP, this synthesis occurring several hours before a transport effect could be seen. The CaBP content of mucosal tissue increased in parallel with the rate of calcium transport. They concluded that vitamin D acted at a transcriptional level, and that CaBP might play a primary role in vitamin D-mediated calcium transport.

This question of the timing of calcium transport and the synthesis of CaBP has been raised by Harmeyer and DeLuca (1969). They found several hours difference in the onset of increased calcium absorption and the appearance of CaBP after vitamin D dosage in both chicks and rats, the calcium absorption rate rising first. While lowering the calcium content of the diet shortened the time lag period of calcium absorption, it had no effect on the time of appearance of CaBP, and they thus concluded that CaBP was not directly related to calcium absorption. However, the results of MacGregor *et al.* (1970), using the much more delicate detection of CaBP synthesis, seem to confirm the general thesis of Wasserman and his group. All the evidence cited above strongly suggests that CaBP plays a major role in calcium transport.

Krawitt and Kunin (1971) examined the mucosa of rats on a high-calcium, low-phosphorus diet which was vitamin D free. Another group was on the same diet but with adequate phosphorus. The first group had rickets, the second did not. Irrespective of these differences, the levels of CaBP were the same in the mucosa of both groups. They concluded that the synthesis of CaBP was independent of dietary phosphate and of the presence of rickets. These results are presumably to be expected since, as will be seen, vitamin D has probably no effect on the absorption of phosphate.

Action of Actinomycin D

It was mentioned above that actinomycin D prevented the appearance of CaBP and the enhanced calcium absorption caused by vitamin D (Corradino and Wasserman, 1968b). Several workers have noted that actinomycin D given to the animal before the intestine was removed would block calcium transport. Norman (1965), studying the time relations in rachitic chicks, found that actinomycin D had to be given before vitamin D for this action to occur. Actinomycin D given 2 hours before vitamin D still blocked the effect of an enormous dose of the vitamin. Zull et al. (1965) reported similar findings and showed that the effect was not due to the inhibition of parathyroid hormone synthesis. Norman (1966) found that within 30 minutes of giving a large dose of vitamin D_3 to rachitic chicks there was considerable synthesis of RNA in the intestinal mucosa; D_2 had no such effect, the synthesis being prevented by actinomycin D. He speculated that the primary effect of vitamin D was to cause RNA and protein synthesis in the mucosal cells. Stohs et al. (1967) gave tritiated orotic acid to D-deficient rats, and reported that within 3 hours of the administration of D_3 there was an incorporation of this purine precursor into RNA, again completely blocked by actinomycin D. It thus appears most probable that calcium absorption is related to the synthesis of a protein, the CaBP of Wasserman.

Enzymes and Calcium Absorption

Martin et al. (1969) and Melancon and DeLuca (1970) described a calcium-dependent ATPase in the brush border of both rat and chick small intestine. On giving vitamin D to D-depleted animals, the content of this enzyme was markedly increased, this increase correlating well with the increase in calcium absorption. On analogy with other organs, where ATPase has been implicated with ion transport, they considered that this enzyme might be involved in calcium transport.

Further work suggests that this enzyme is associated with alkaline phosphatase. Norman *et al.* (1970) found that alkaline phosphatase was increased in the mucosa at the same time that calcium transport was stimulated by vitamin D. Haussler *et al.* (1970) noted an increase in both calcium-dependent ATPase activity and alkaline phosphatase when vitamin D was given to rachitic chicks, and from inhibition studies concluded that both enzymes were properties of the same enzyme molecule. Holdsworth (1970) also concluded that calcium-dependent ATPase activity resided in an alkaline phosphatase; although this enzyme could be inhibited by *dl*-phenylalanine, this amino acid has no effect upon calcium transport. Thus the exact role of this enzyme system in calcium absorption has not been elucidated.

Vitamin D affects other ions besides calcium and will increase the absorption of several other, but necessarily physiological cations, e.g., barium, magnesium, beryllium, strontium (Worker and Migicovsky, 1961a,b; Wasserman, 1962).

Phosphorus Absorption

There seems to be some question as to whether the vitamin also affects phosphorus absorption. Older workers such as Dols *et al.* (1937) and Morgareidge and Manley (1939), using the then recently available radiophosphorus, found no evidence that vitamin D controlled phosphorus absorption. Harrison and Harrison (1961) reported that phosphorus was absorbed against a concentration gradient, this being inhibited by cyanide or anaerobiosis. Calcium had to be present and EDTA treatment completely inhibited phosphorus transport. Intestines of vitamin D-deficient rats concentrated phosphorus less well than those of vitamin D-treated animals, but this vitamin effect was abolished when calcium was removed. Kowarski and Schachter (1969) studied the problem both *in vitro* and *in vivo*. In the case of *in vitro* experiments, they found that previous dosage with vitamin D increased the transfer of phosphorus from mucosa to serosa in rachitic rats.

Closed loops were used *in vivo*, and the vitamin was put directly into them. Phosphorus absorption was again increased, the vitamin thus acting without prior activation by other organs. On the other hand, Sallis and Holdsworth (1962) found that under conditions when vitamin D could increase calcium transport threefold in rachitic chicks, it had no action on the transport of phosphorus.

Both Thompson and DeLuca (1964) and Neville and Holdsworth (1968) have reported that vitamin D increased the incorporation of radioactive phosphorus into phospholipids (and also into acid-soluble phosphorus and ATP) of the mucosa, provided calcium was also present. The total amount of phospholipids was not increased and the vitamin had no effect upon phospholipid metabolism, but in the presence of calcium there was increased phosphorus translocation and thus augmentation in the specific activity of phosphorus compounds in the mucosa.

It seems that all these effects, many of which are calcium dependent, are due to the transfer of phosphorus with calcium, and the increased specific activity of the lipids was due to the increased amount of label presented to them. The evidence that vitamin D has a specific effect on phosphorus absorption alone is not strong.

Submicroscopic Location of Vitamin D

It has been possible, using labeled vitamin D, to determine with which submicroscopic fraction of the mucosa the vitamin is associated. Haussler and Norman (1967) gave tritiated vitamin D_3 to rachitic chicks and found that the nuclei of the mucosa accumulated a large portion of the dose, the same being found if homogenates of small intestine were incubated with the vitamin. Stohs and DeLuca (1967) reported vitamin D and its metabolites to be associated with the nuclear membrane of the mucosa, 80% being in a biologically active form. Wilson *et al.* (1967) reported similar findings, the vitamin being found in highest concentration in a fraction consisting of brush borders and nuclei. In vitamin D-deficient rats, the microsomal fraction contained more vitamin D than that of mitochondria, but after vitamin D dosage the content of each was equal, appreciable metabolism of vitamin D occurred, and the metabolites were found predominantly in the mitochondrial fraction. Haussler *et al.* (1968), after giving labeled vitamin D, detected radioactivity associated with a nuclear chromatin fraction, largely as a polar metabolite. This association could be competitively inhibited by cold vitamin D_3, D_2, or dihydrotachysterol. Chen *et al.* (1970) criticized the method used by these workers, maintaining that this fractionation included membranes and cell organelles; Chen's group adhered to the view (expressed above) by the DeLuca school that only membranes were involved.

Sampson *et al.* (1970) used ^{45}Ca in an electron microscopic study. They found calcium in the microvilli and mitochondria of normal animals, but the granules were very sparse in the mitochondria of vitamin D-deficient animals. They thought vitamin D to be necessary for the release of calcium bound in the microvilli, whence it progressed to mitochondria, or through the cell to the circulation. But in animals with adequate vitamin D or deficient in the vitamin, calcium granules were absorbed across the cellular membrane and bound within the microvilli.

The germfree state increased intestinal calcium absorption but did not affect that of phosphorus. Calcium and phosphorus retention were increased (Reddy *et al.*, 1969).

Vitamin D Metabolites

In 1944 Irving noted that the vitamin required a definite length of time before it began to act on the skeleton. He studied the response in the incisor teeth of rachitic rats where it is possible to measure the time of action of vitamin D upon dentin recalcification and suggested that "a certain state" had to occur in the body before the vitamin became active. He further noted that the time of action was inversely proportional to the logarithm of the dose of vitamin D, physiological dose levels being used. Coates and Holdsworth (1961) narrowed down the time of action as they found that vitamin D given to chicks would increase calcium absorption if given 16 hours before, but had no effect if given less than 8 hours before.

It was not possible at that time, because of the lack of microchemical methods, to proceed further, and it was not till 1967 that Morii *et al.* isolated a new metabolite of vitamin D_3 from rats. This was as effective as vitamin D in healing rickets, raising blood calcium, and increasing calcium transport in everted sacs, and acted much more quickly than did vitamin D. Blunt *et al.* (1968) isolated and identified an active metabolite of vitamin D_3 from the plasma of pigs fed large doses of vitamin D_3. This was found to be 25-hydroxycholecalciferol (25-HCC), and it was found to be 1.4 times as effective as vitamin D_3 in curing rickets in rats. They postulated that this was the active form of the vitamin. Blunt and DeLuca (1969) synthesized 25-HCC and found that when given to the animals before sacrifice it was much quicker in stimulating calcium transport in everted sacs. Olsen and DeLuca (1969) perfused intestinal loops of vitamin D-deficient rats *in situ* through both the lumen and the circulation. On adding 25-HCC to the arterial blood, within 2 hours calcium transport was raised to the same level as that of rats which had been given vitamin D before sacrifice; vitamin D_3 put into the arterial circulation had no such effect. Thus 25-HCC had a local effect which vitamin D did not possess.

Ponchon and DeLuca (1969) cited experiments which suggested that the liver was the major site of transformation of vitamin D_3 into 25-HCC. Chicks could apparently change both D_2 and D_3 into the active polar form, but the metabolite from vitamin D_2 had but little action on chicks (Drescher *et al.*, 1969). The transformation into a polar metabolite was shown by Avioli *et al.* (1967) to have possible clinical implications; they found that in vitamin D-resistant rickets and familial hypophosphatasia there was a decrease in the conversion of vitamin D into a polar biologically active metabolite.

25-Hydroxyergocalciferol was isolated from pig blood, identified as the active metabolite of vitamin D_2 (Suda *et al.*, 1969), and was found to be 1.5 times as active in curing rickets in rats as was D_2 or D_3. An interesting implication arises from all these findings. Suda *et al.* say that "there is now mounting evidence that vitamin D_3 [cholecalciferol] must be converted into its metabolically active form before it can produce its characteristic physiological response." This implies that vitamin D_2 or D_3 as such are inactive. Thus comparisons of the activities of these vitamins with that of their metabolites merely reflect their degree of conversion into such metabolites. If the metabolite was 1.5 times as active as the original vitamin, the conversion was at most about 66%, the rest of the vitamin being either excreted unchanged or converted into inactive compounds.

There are undoubtedly other active vitamin D metabolites. Suda *et al.* (1970a,b) have described two dihydroxylated cholecalciferol derivatives that have some vitamin D activity. Cousins *et al.* (1970) considered that 25-HCC was the circulating or hormonal form of vitamin D, and that this gave rise to regulatory forms which acted in bone or on the intestine.

Other workers, however, have cast doubt on the importance of 25-HCC as the metabolically active form of vitamin D_3. The two chief groups are those of Kodicek and Norman. Lawson *et al.* (1969a,b) reported that the active metabolite they isolated from intestinal cell nuclei was not 25-HCC, but was probably formed from it. In their most recent paper, Lawson *et al.* (1971) identified this compound as 1,25-dihydroxycholecalciferol (1,25-DHCC). It was formed in the kidney and was to be regarded as a hormone controlling calcium metabolism. It was twice as active as cholecalciferol in stimulating calcium absorption, and accumulated in the target tissues, bone, and the mucosal cell nuclei of the small intestine. Vitamin D thus resembled the steroid hormones "in the changes it brings about in the template capacity of the DNA and in RNA synthesis in its target tissues."

Norman and his group report the same. Myrtle *et al.* (1970) described a compound 4B, bound to intestinal chromatin, which was not 25-HCC. The metabolite was made in the kidney from 25-HCC (Norman *et al.*, 1971a), was more than 4 times as active as cholecalciferol, twice as active as 25-HCC in stimulating calcium absorption in rachitic chicks, and acted much faster than either. In their most recent paper, Norman *et al.* (1971b) have confirmed that their compound 4B was in fact 1, 25-DHCC.

It is of interest that Avioli *et al.* (1969b) found that in experimental renal failure in rats, the activity of CaBP was reduced. This activity could not be increased by vitamin D_3, but was increased by giving 25-HCC.

Corradino and Wasserman (1970a) cite an example in which vitamin D can act directly on the intestine, and does not require the intervention of a remote tissue. Surviving embryo chick intestine, in organ culture, formed CaBP when either vitamin D_3 or 25-HCC was added to the medium.

It is difficult at this stage to assess these various reports on vitamin D metabolites. One question has definitely been answered: The delay in vitamin D action is due to the time taken to convert it into an active form. As to which is this active form, only future research can decide. For some time, it was believed to be 25-HCC. Now a new metabolite with more rapid and greater activity has been described, and possibly before long still more active polar metabolites will be found. It seems, however, reasonable to conclude that a chain reaction occurs: Vitamin D is changed into active forms that may act at the transcriptional level on the mucosal cell, thereby stimulating the production of a calcium-carrying protein, which transports calcium across the cell, and may have actions on other target cells.

There seems to be further implications in these findings. Nicolaysen (1943) had suggested that the intestinal absorption of calcium was a function of the calcium saturation of the body and that this was governed by an endogenous factor which needed vitamin D for it to act. It is possible that the rate of calcium loss from the body and not its calcium saturation is the factor that controls calcium absorption in the intestine. The kidney's production of 1,25-DHCC may be sensitive to the level of calcium loss and might thus control by humoral means, the rate of calcium absorption.

Distribution of Vitamin D in the Body

Kodicek and Ashley (1960) were among the first to prepare labeled vitamin D. They gave it orally in small and large amounts to normal and rachitic rats and followed the fate of the label in the body. In most cases the biological activity of the label decreased significantly. Twenty-four hours later, the bulk of the radioactivity was in the feces, more being present in the excreta of the rachitic animals. The liver took up about 8% of the dose. The rachitic intestinal tissue took up 2.0%, that of normal animals having only 0.5%. The bones had a small activity. When the vitamin was given intracardially (Kodicek *et al.*, 1960), the distribution differed in that much activity accumulated in the liver. Imrie *et al.* (1967) gave tritiated vitamin D_3 to chicks and found a high concentration of activity in bone cells and intestinal mucosa, and DeLuca *et al.* (1968), using a vitamin D derivative ($[22–23^3H] D_4$), also noted a high content in bone cells and intestinal mucosa. The liver had a high content of the label initially, but released it quite rapidly. This was probably due to its transformation into active metabolites and sub-sequent discharge into the bloodstream. Holman *et al.* (1970) also studied the distribution of labeled vitamin D_3 in rats, and found there were three areas of vitamin retention. The liver and plasma had a high retention at first, but this fell rapidly. Some tissues had a slower accumulation and decline; these were the intestinal mucosa, kidney, bone, and muscle. Last, adipose tissue had a slowly increasing content and no decline. In the liver, plasma, and intestinal mucosa, 80% of the activity was present after 1 week as a more polar metabolite. Thus in general the radioactivity was found where it would be expected, in organs known to be influenced by vitamin D. It is surprising that the liver stored so little of the vitamin.

Vitamin D was associated in the bloodstream with globulin, probably α-globulin (Rikkers and DeLuca, 1967); the binding was specific for vitamin D_3 and more effective than the binding of D_2 or D_4. Addition of a hydroxy group to the vitamins increased their affinity for the protein (Rikkers *et al.*, 1969). More recently Haddad and Chyu (1971) reported that 85% of 25-HCC was bound to an inter-α-globulin, and 10% was associated with albumin. The molecular weight of the binding protein was 40,000–50,000, and cholecalciferol and ergocalciferol were less competitive in protein binding. Mawer and Stanbury (1968) gave labeled cholecalciferol intravenously to humans. They found that the radioactivity of a polar metabolite in the blood rose from zero and reached a maximum within 7–14 days, and then decayed with a long half-life. Thus vitamin D was retained in the bloodstream as polar metabolites longer than previously supposed.

_____ *Chapter 3*

INTESTINAL ABSORPTION
OF CALCIUM AND PHOSPHORUS
Data from Balance Experiments

Calcium

It has long been known that the absorption of calcium in the human intestine is by no means complete, although in other species the process may be more efficient. Much work has been done on the availability of various forms of calcium. One of the most recent reports is that of Nordin *et al.* (1964), who found that ^{47}Ca administered as chloride was more readily absorbed then when it was given as orthophosphate, glycerophosphate, carbonate, or in milk. Whittemore and Thompson (1969) devised a new way of determining the availability of calcium or phosphorus by comparing the total body retention after oral or parenteral administration of ^{4r}Ca or ^{32}P. A comparison of these figures with those obtained by balance experiments showed that this method was valid; the analysis could in fact be limited to a single bone and thus used in large animals. Provided the calcium is soluble or can be made soluble as, for example, by the hydrochloric acid of the gastric juice, it is available for absorption in some degree. As is well known, bone meal is commonly given to farm animals. In general, plant calcium is less available than that from animal sources (Breiter *et al.*, 1942).

Much work has been done on the degree of absorption of dietary calcium and phosphorus. Earlier work, in which it was assumed that this figure could be arrived at by subtracting the fecal value from the intake, took no account of the endogenous loss, although Bergeim as early as 1926 had pointed out that both calcium and phosphorus entered and left the intestine at various levels. This endogenous loss of calcium and phosphorus arises from these elements inside the body, which are returned to the gut lumen in the intestinal secretions. Little is known of the factors controlling this process, but by the use of labeled calcium or phosphorus it has been possible to estimate the level of loss.

IN ANIMALS

Studies in rats showed a very high calcium absorption when the animals were on low calcium intakes, the absorption rate falling as the intake of calcium rose (Hansard and Plumlee, 1954). The percentage absorption of calcium fell with age in rats (Hansard and Crowder, 1957) but as the total intake rose with age, the absolute amount of calcium absorbed did not change much. Hironaka *et al.* (1960) also found an age difference in rats, in that older animals absorbed more calcium and had a higher endogenous loss than younger ones. They considered the higher calcium absorption to be an adaptive mechanism to maintain calcium equilibrium. Sammon *et al.* (1970) found the levels of calcium intake and endogenous loss to vary directly.

The calcium absorption of cows has been studied by Hansard and his group (1954) and as with rats, the percentage absorption fell with age. Smith (1962) fistulated calves and reported that up to the end of the small intestine the mean net absorption of calcium was about 86%, and decreased with age. There was a negligible calcium exchange in the large intestine.

Lueker and Lofgreen (1961) investigated the absorption of calcium and phosphorus in lambs on diets with different Ca:P ratios. The various ratios had no effect on the amount of labeled calcium or phosphorus absorbed, which was governed solely by the amount of the element fed. Metabolic fecal calcium was the same with all dietary ratios, but the metabolic fecal phosphorus increased as the phosphorus absorbed increased. Very similar findings were reported by Young *et al.* (1966) working with sheep.

Singer *et al.* (1957), in short-term investigations with dogs, injected ^{45}Ca intravenously, and found 50% of the endogenous excretion within the small intestine, and 40% in the large intestine.

In Humans

Brine and Johnston (1955) summarized the figures in the literature for humans up to that date. They calculated the fecal endogenous loss in adults to be about 75 mg/day, and as the calcium intake rose from 400 to 1200 mg/day the percentage absorption fell from 43 to 28%. Blau et al. (1957) studied 2 elderly patients with ^{45}Ca, using the method of isotope dilution. The endogenous fecal loss was about 100 mg/day and was independent of the dietary calcium level. The total digestive juice calcium was quite different in the two subjects, 150 mg/day in one, and 360 mg in the other, and was also independent of the calcium intake; 45–65% of the dietary calcium was absorbed.

Lutwak and Shapiro (1964) conducted a large volume liquid scintillation counter study on a human and found absorption of 59 and 67% in two separate experiments. Parsons et al. (1968) gave ^{47}Ca to humans aged 26–66 with a total calcium intake around 1000 mg/day. The calcium absorption was from 15 to 34%, and bore no relation to the calcium intake, nor to the age of the patients. The urinary excretion was variable and had no relation to the intake; the endogenous loss was also variable, averaging about 300 mg/day. Calcium absorption correlated with the blood and fecal data once allowance was made for the endogenous secretion. They found the 2-hour plasma activity of radioactive calcium to correlate fairly well with the degree of calcium absorption, an index originally introduced by Bhandarkar et al. (1961).

Thus in animals in general the percentage calcium absorption drops with age, but there are not sufficient data to state whether the absolute amount of calcium retained changes very much. In all species it appears that the endogenous loss is independent of the calcium intake. This is to be expected, since the rate of secretion of intestinal juices is probably not controlled at all by the dietary calcium.

There seems to be a species difference in the relative excretion of calcium in the urine and feces. Wanner et al. (1956) injected ^{45}Ca into a number of animals. Monkeys and men had a relatively low fecal excretion compared to rats and dogs, since the primates excreted twice as much radioactive calcium in the urine compared to feces, the other animals losing much more in the feces.

Hart and Spencer (1967), working with humans, studied the rate of entry of ^{47}Ca from the intestine into the vascular space. The maximum rate was reached in 1.5 hours, was sustained for about 1 hour, and then declined, by which time about 20–40% of the dose had been absorbed. Finally, after 7.5 hours, 30–59% had been absorbed. In 1966 Samachson *et al.* had found that in a given subject the degree of radioactive calcium absorption was the same at all times of the day, the percentage absorbed being inversely proportional to the level of calcium intake.

Habituation to Low Calcium Intakes

It has long been known that during habituation to low calcium diets calcium absorption is increased. Luick *et al.* (1957) found that cows adjusted to changes in calcium and phosphorus intake by changing the degree of absorption rather than by altering the endogenous loss. Kimberg *et al.* (1961), using rats, reported that calcium deprivation increased active transport most in the duodenum, vitamin D being necessary for this to occur. This response to low calcium diets was unaffected by thyroparathyroidectomy, hypophysectomy, or adrenalectomy. Gran (1960) had reported the same as far as the parathyroid was concerned. Finkelstein and Schachter (1962), however, found active transport to be decreased in everted sacs from hypophysectomized rats, the effect being reversed by previous treatment with growth hormone; the same was found *in vivo*. Shah and Draper (1966) considered that the parathyroid gland was involved in adaptation to low calcium diets, but Sammon *et al.* (1970) were unable to confirm their findings, and reported that only at high levels of calcium intake did parathyroidectomy lead to a decrease in calcium absorption. Harrison and Harrison (1960) reported that cortisol administration induced active transport in everted sacs and thought that it influenced the permeability of cell surfaces to calcium.

This somewhat confused story is related to Nicolaysen's hypothesis (1943) that the intestinal absorption of calcium was a function of the calcium saturation of the body and was governed by an endogenous factor, which needed vitamin D for its action. Further evidence for this concept was provided by Haavaldsen and Nicolaysen (1956). Gran (1960), on the basis of his findings, did not consider the endogenous factor to be parathyroid hormone. As described elsewhere, low calcium diets have an effect on the calcium absorptive mechanism at the molecular level and the evidence suggests that this action is a direct one on mucosal cells. Nicolaysen's factor may be a vitamin D metabolite.

Other Factors Affecting Calcium Absorption

Much work has been done showing that in experimental animals the fat level of the diet can influence calcium absorption. The question is probably of academic importance as far as healthy humans are concerned, except possibly in the case of infants, since, for example, Filer and Foman (1967) have reported that when newborn infants retain fat poorly, calcium is also poorly retained. Mallon *et al.* (1930) and Steggerda and Mitchell (1951) found that dietary fat over a wide range had no effect upon calcium retention in humans. Humans do not normally eat fat-free diets, or diets with a fat content over 20%.

Bile acids have been implicated in calcium absorption. Lengemann and Dobbins (1958) reported that an increased bile flow enhanced calcium absorption. Webling and Holdsworth (1965) worked with normal and rachitic chicks and found that chick bile caused an immediate increase in calcium absorption, which they attributed to an anionic detergent action of bile acids. They assumed this to be the explanation since sodium lauryl sulfate, an anionic detergent, was also found to be effective. On the other hand, cationic detergents had no such effect, and they considered that anionic detergents formed salts or complexes, soluble to some extent in both aqueous and lipid phases. In a later paper (1966) they reported that bile acids increased the solubility of calcium in lipid solvents to approximately the same extent that they increased calcium absorption.

In 1956 Wasserman *et al.* reported that several amino acids promoted calcium absorption. Radioactive calcium was used, and deposition in the femur 24 hours later was taken as the measure of absorption. The amino acids had to be given at the same time as the labeled calcium, lysine and arginine being the most effective. Solubility of the compounds was not the cause of the better absorption, since calcium–glycine was very soluble, but glycine was not particularly effective. Both D- and L-lysine were equal in their ability to increase calcium absorption. L-Lysine promoted calcium absorption in rachitic rats, as did vitamin D, and both together had an additive effect (Wasserman *et al.*, 1957a). Raven *et al.* (1960) showed, by ligating segments of the small intestine, that lysine had to be in the same segment as calcium and that the effect was most marked in the ileum.

Another compound that improves calcium absorption is lactose. It has been known for some time that this sugar improved calcium retention and could alleviate parathyroid tetany (McCullagh and McCullagh, 1932). Fournier (1954) felt that lactose plays a specific and important role in calcium metabolism. Wasserman and his group have studied this phenomenon in some detail. In 1956 (Wasserman *et al.*, 1956) they reported that lactose had a stronger effect than lysine and that the effect was additive if given with lysine (Wasserman *et al.*, 1957a). As with lysine, lactose had to be given at the same time as calcium, and be in the same segment of the intestine. Its action was local in the intestine, since if it was given intraperitoneally, no effect was seen. Nor was the effect due to the development of a special intestinal flora (Lengemann, 1959). Lengemann *et al.* (1959) also found that lactose would promote calcium absorption in rachitic rats, both in the presence and absence of vitamin D, and was as effective in this regard as vitamin D itself. The action was not due to acids produced by bacteria, and it was, as with lysine, most marked in the ileum, though it was also seen in the duodenum and jejunum.

Wasserman and Comar (1959) stated that some other carbohydrates had an action similar to that of lactose, but they were ones that stayed for some time in the intestinal lumen (cellobiose, sorbose, ribose, xylose, and lactose), but carbohydrates that were rapidly absorbed had little or no effect. They thought the lactose effect was a nonspecific membrane phenomenon, increasing permeability not only to calcium but also to other alkali earth cations (Wasserman and Lengemann, 1960). It seemed very unlikely that a Ca–lactose complex was formed, since after the ingestion of radioactive lactose all areas of the intestine were equally labeled with ^{14}C, but the lactose effect was restricted predominantly to the ileum (Lengemann and Comar, 1963). No explanation of the effects of lactose or lysine has been forthcoming.

Various other factors, such as pH of the intestinal content, bulk of diet, and acidosis, have been alleged to play a role in calcium absorption. The literature was reviewed by Irving (1957), who considered that under normal conditions these factors played no significant role in this regard. There appears to be two processes of calcium absorption—active and passive. We do not know at present the relative importance of each.

Absorption of Phosphorus

The absorption of phosphorus has been much less investigated. Cramer (1959), working with normal rats, investigated the radioactivity of the tail after administering ^{32}P. Absorption was very rapid, the peak being reached in 30 minutes. Dymsza *et al.* (1959) fed high or low levels of ortho- or metaphosphate to rats and found no effect upon absorption of calcium or phosphorus. Hevesy (1948) determined that with daily phosphorus intakes of about 1400 mg, the human fecal endogenous loss was about 24–31% of the intake.

It seems possible from some of the earlier work (Artom *et al.*, 1938; Fries *et al.*, 1938) that a major part of ^{32}P intake by mouth was incorporated into phospholipids in the intestinal wall, which is probably a reflection of the synthesis of lipids from absorbed fats.

Phytic acid or inositol hexaphosphoric acid is found as a large part of the organic phosphorus of cereals and seeds, partly in the free state, and partly as phytin, the calcium magnesium salt. Its significance as far as calcium metabolism is concerned is that it forms an insoluble salt with calcium and thus may interfere with calcium absorption in the intestine. Animal experiments have shown that it can interfere with calcium absorption, but this has never been convincingly demonstrated in man. Some animals have a phytase in their intestinal secretions, but no such enzyme has been demonstrated in man. However, during baking a substantial amount of phytic acid is hydrolyzed by phytase in the flour, and the yeast in the dough also has this enzyme, which can act while the dough is standing.

Experiments carried out in England on humans during World War II seemed to indicate that bread made from high extraction flours contained enough phytic acid to slowly demineralize the skeleton, and as a result chalk was compulsorily added to the national wheatmeal during the war and after it was over. Walker *et al.* (1948) did long-term balance experiments on humans who ate bread made from almost straight-run flour. They found that there was an initial negative calcium balance, but that subsequently adaptation occurred, and positive calcium balances were attained. They criticized conclusions drawn from the results of short-term balance experiments, when no chance of adaptation could occur. The consensus of opinion is that on diets habitually eaten by humans, there is no danger at all from anticalcifying factors in cereals (Bronner *et al.*, 1956).

_____ *Chapter 4*

CALCIUM AND PHOSPHORUS CONTENT OF THE BODY

Total Calcium

This has been investigated in animals, chiefly rats, by a number of workers. Unfortunately, in the case of man, few and discrepant figures are available; very few indeed in the case of children, and many unreliable ones in the case of adults.

IN ANIMALS

The newborn rat is virtually calcium-free. Cox and Imboden (1936) found that a newborn rat weighing 5 g contained about 14 mg calcium. At weaning (21 days) and weighing 48 g, it contained 313 mg calcium. The mineral content at weaning was fairly constant and females contained more calcium than males. Bessey *et al.* (1935) found that 99.06% of the total calcium was in the skeleton and teeth at 2 months of age and 99.3% at 4 months.

A more recent study of the calcium content of the animal body was made by Spray and Widdowson (1950). In the case of rats, they found that a large increase in calcium content occurred during the suckling period, after which the rate of accretion gradually fell until the mature percentage was reached; this occurred in the rat at about 100 days. A kink in the curve of accretion at about 30 days was presumably due to new feeding conditions following weaning. The Ca:P weight ratio of the body was 0.91 for the male rat at birth and rose gradually to 1.75 at 246 days of age. The calcium content of adult male rats was about 1.1% and of females about 1.3% in whole, fat-free body tissues. Saville and Smith (1966) reported that the total body calcium and the calcium content of individual long bones of the rat were a linear function of the body weight in both sexes: the total skeletal calcium a constant percentage of the weight in males, but a continuously increasing percentage of the body weight in females.

Spray and Widdowson also gave figures for the rabbit, cat, pig, and mouse. The accretion figures for rat, mouse, and rabbit are similar and all begin life with a very low calcium content. The sex difference in the rat is not seen in the rabbit. The calcium content of the fat-free body of piglets fell sharply from birth to day 7, after which it rose steadily (Manners and McCrea, 1963).

Effects of Dietary Calcium

A great deal of work has been done on the effect of dietary and other factors upon the calcium content of the body—most of the work being done on rats. The composition of the newborn rat is remarkably constant despite changes in the mother's diet (Goss and Schmidt, 1930); but if the mother's diet is poor, many more young are born dead. With drastic changes in the mother, such as giving her a very high Ca:P ratio diet after parathyroidectomy, the fetal calcium and phosphorus are lowered, while giving vitamin D to the mother improved the fetal storage of calcium and phosphorus (Bodansky and Duff, 1941).

Most work on the effects of the calcium content of the diet upon that of the body was done by Sherman and his colleagues and almost entirely on rats. Animals on low calcium diets and stunted in growth, had total calcium contents higher than that of animals of corresponding weight, but lower than that of animals of corresponding age (Sherman and Macleod, 1925). If the calcium intake was very low, the body calcium remained stationary and the animals lived for about 6 weeks, showing at the end of that time multiple calcium deficiencies, but not rickets. Addition of calcium to such a diet increased the body percentage to the right figure, though the absolute amount was too low and the animals now had rickets. Campbell *et al.* (1935) found that the second-generation of rats on a poor calcium diet (0.094%) could survive but could not reproduce and had only 75–80% of the normal total calcium content of the body. The addition of phosphorus as potassium phosphate to a low calcium diet accelerated calcium uptake so that it was actually higher in percentage than the normal figure for that age though still low in absolute amount (Sherman and Pappenheimer, 1921). With a fixed dietary phosphorus content of 0.43%, increasing the calcium up to 1.04% had no effect upon the body calcium, but if the phosphorus was fixed at 0.73%, the calcium content of the body was increased by extra dietary calcium (Whitcher *et al.*, 1936). Shohl *et al.* (1933) found in much the same way that the phosphorus intake was a limiting factor in the control of the calcium content of the body in the rat.

Sherman and Booher (1931) investigated growing animals on diets containing 0.16–0.50% calcium. Although all the animals grew at the same rate and looked equally healthy, those on the higher calcium intake contained more calcium during the growth period, the difference gradually disappearing as the rats became middle-aged. In a later paper (Lanford *et al.*, 1941) it was shown that rats on a diet containing 0.64% calcium reached a level of total body calcium which was not attained by rats on a diet with 0.35% calcium till 50 days later. Fairbanks and Mitchell (1936) also found that the carcass calcium increased with high calcium contents of the diet.

It thus appears that the total calcium content of the body can be increased by extra calcium in the diet during growth even though the growth rate and appearance of the animals are unaffected.

Placental Transfer of Calcium and Phosphorus

The literature on this is somewhat conflicting. Feaster *et al.* (1956) found that ^{45}Ca easily traversed the rat placenta and was deposited in the fetus within 30 minutes of giving it to the mother. The opposite movement could not occur according to Payne and Sansom (1963). They gave the mother rats severe hypocalcemia with EDTA and found that ^{47}Ca injected into the fetus did not return to the mother. However, the placenta could not compensate for calcium deficiency in the mother by delivering the normal amount of calcium to the fetus under these circumstances. Bawden and McIver (1964) found in calcium-deficient rats that the ratio of uptake of ^{45}Ca by the fetus was the same as that in the maternal femur, in both normal and deficient states.

In guinea pigs a rather different picture is seen. Hypercalcemia, brought about in the mother by parathyroid extract, vitamin D, or calcium infusions, did not elevate the fetal plasma calcium (Burnette *et al.*, 1968; Greeson *et al.*, 1968). Twardock and Austin (1970) perfused the guinea pig placenta and concluded that there was active calcium transfer and that diffusion of calcium did not occur.

In pigs, ^{45}Ca went easily across the placenta (Shirley *et al.*, 1954). The rate of ^{32}P transfer in these animals was directly related to fetal size, and rose steadily during the last half of pregnancy.

MacDonald *et al.* (1965), working with rhesus monkeys, injected ^{45}Ca into the maternal, and ^{47}Ca into the fetal, circulation, and determined them simultaneously. They found a two-way exchange, the amount of calcium crossing the placenta being 6 to 10 times the amount required for fetal skeletal growth.

There does not seem to be much relationship between the structure of these various placentas and their handling of calcium. Primates, rats, and guinea pigs have a hemochorial placenta, in which the maternal endothelium has been lost, and transmission should be most rapid and complete (Hansel and McEntee, 1970). This seems to be the case for the rat and rhesus, but does not apply to the guinea pig. The pig placenta is of the epitheliochorial type, with six tissue layers separating the maternal and fetal blood, and is the most primitive of placentas. In spite of this apparent structural barrier, calcium and phosphorus appear to traverse it easily.

Kronfeld *et al.* (1971) have carried out kinetic analyses of placental calcium transfer in monkeys and sheep, and have calculated the rate of active transport in the two species. In spite of the difference in size of the fetuses, the active transport rates on a weight basis were quite similar. The net diffusion of calcium from fetus to mother was relatively much greater in the monkey than the sheep, possibly due to differences in placental structure, as the sheep placenta is of the epitheliochorial type.

Experiments with pregnant rabbits and rats have shown that when

[45]Ca and ^{32}P were injected, the amount of calcium and phosphorus reaching the fetuses was just about enough to meet their requirements (Wilde *et al.*, 1946; Wasserman *et al.*, 1957b). Wilde *et al.* found that fetal guinea pigs and rats incorporated into their bodies all the calcium and inorganic phosphorus in the mother's serum every hour, but Widdowson (1962) has reported for the human fetus, which grows more slowly, that only 5% of the calcium and 10% of the inorganic phosphorus of the mother's plasma is so used.

Calcium Content in Humans

IN UTERO FIGURE

Fehling (1877) was the first to analyze fetuses. Since then many more analyses have been made and more recent figures have been reported by Coons (1935), Iob and Swanson (1934), and Givens and Macy (1933). The latter authors found the calcium content to rise in an apparently exponential way, when plotted against age, to a final calcium content of 21 g at term, the greatest calcium demand coming in the last 3 months of gestation. The most recent and authoritative findings are those of Widdowson and Spray (1951), who analyzed fetuses and stillborn children weighing from 200 g to 4.4 kg. The total calcium rose continually from about 2 g at the first weight to 36 g at 4.4 kg body weight, the rise being linear when plotted against body weight after the fetus weighed 0.4 kg. The percentage of calcium likewise rose, but more slowly from 0.4% to 1.0% on a fat-free body basis.

IN GROWING CHILDREN

Knowledge of the calcium content of the body of the child during growth is of importance in assessing the dietary calcium requirements of children, but little direct information exists on this subject. Many attempts have been made to compute figures, based on the calcium content of the newborn child, that of the adult, and various assumptions on the rate of accretion of calcium during various phases of the growth process. There is no point in mentioning these attempts as they are now solely of historical interest. However, in 1945 Mitchell and his colleagues reported analyses of a fresh male cadaver and obtained a figure for total body calcium of 1.596%. On the basis of this more accurate figure for the adult calcium content, these workers reassessed the estimate of the daily calcium increments during growth. The growth data of Meredith (1941) were used, and these assumptions were made: (a) The calcium content at birth is 0.8% (whole body basis); (b) that in the adult is 1.6%; (c) the change from the infantile to the adult percentage occurs progressively during growth, but more rapidly when growth is more rapid, and thus the calcium gains were greatest over the period of 14–18 years; the final assumption was based upon findings with growing rats, chickens, and lambs, and it appeared valid to apply them to humans.

Some of the calculated figures for body calcium are shown in the following tabulation.

Age	Weight (kg)	Ca content (g)
1	10.6	100
5	19.1	219
10	33.3	396
15	55.0	806
20	67.0	1078

Widdowson et al. (1951) analyzed the body of a boy aged 4.5 years who died of tuberculous meningitis after a 2-week illness. The body was moderately nourished but rather thin and weighed 14 kg. The calcium content was given as a percentage of the fat-free body and on recalculation the total calcium is found to be 228 g. The weight of the boy was considerably less than that given by Mitchell and his group (17.6 kg at 4 years and 19.1 kg at 5 years), and the calcium content was higher than Mitchell's (219 g at 5 years). Unfortunately, it is impossible to draw any reliable conclusions from one analysis and that of the body of a very ill child.

IN THE ADULT

Here too it must be admitted that while figures from cadaver analyses exist, many of them are quite unreliable and the subjects analyzed were not normal. The uncertainty about exact figures has been illustrated by Mitchell et al. (1945), who quote those given in the various editions of Sherman's "Chemistry of Food and Nutrition," the values varying from 1.15 to 2.2%.

Nicholls and Nimalasuriya (1939) analyzed bones from Ceylonese skeletons and arrived at a body calcium figure of 1.65% for males. More recently three analyses have been carried out by Mitchell and his colleagues (Mitchell et al., 1945; Forbes et al., 1953, 1956). These were all estimations of apparently normal males, and the calcium content of the fat-free body varied between 1.8 and 2.5%, the skeleton being from 14.84 to 17.58% of the total body weight, and containing about 99% of the total body calcium. Widdowson et al. (1951) also analyzed the bodies of two men and one woman. The males were not normal but the calcium content of the bodies agreed with the figures of Mitchell's group, being about 2.3% on a fat-free basis. The figures quoted by Sherman seem to be more accurate than was realized.

Calcium Content of Individual Tissues

A bare recital of the calcium content of various tissues is not very informative although calcium plays an essential role in many tissue functions. It will be seen from the following figures that in most cases the calcium level appears to be related to that of the plasma but is not affected much by fluctuations in the plasma level. The exact state of tissue calcium is not known but it would appear to be bound in some fairly stable way (Joseph et al., 1953).

Katz (1896) was the first to give accurate figures for tissue calcium, 7.5 mg/100 g for human muscle and 6.9 mg for dog muscle. Burns (1933) found that of rat muscle to be about 7 mg/100 g; she also gave figures for other rat tissues and muscles of other animals. Rat fat has a very small content, but the brain has values of 8–16 mg/100 g. Dog and cat muscle calcium was of the same order as that of rat; frog muscle has 11–25 mg/100 g. The trachea contains 0.5–4 mg/100 g, the value increasing with age because of calcification of the cartilages. The calcium content of skin has been determined by Brown (1926). The values per 100 g dry skin were highest for the rabbit (50–86 mg) and lowest for the dog and man (31–59 mg).

Bürger and Schlomka (1939) found that the calcium content of the human aorta rose with age from 0.05 g/100 g dry weight at 6.7 years to

1.6 g/100 g at 76 years. Widdowson *et al.* (1951) found that the calcium of human liver was about 6 mg/100 g fresh weight and that of the spleen to be about 9 mg/100 g fresh weight.

Bradbury *et al.* (1968), using atomic absorption flame photometry, obtained results on the whole lower than those reported in the earlier work, in estimations using a number of animals. Skeletal muscle contained 3.2–5.8 mg/100 g and brain 3.9–5.8. The cerebrospinal fluid had 5.2–6 mg/100 ml. The method they used is probably much more accurate and the best available today.

The effect of various factors on the calcium content of tissues has been investigated by several workers. Burns (1933) found no change in muscle calcium after the animals had subsisted on high Ca:P ratio diets, with and without vitamin D, or on low Ca:P ratio diets. The blood calcium was lowered by a variety of means but the muscle calcium remained unchanged. Injections of parathyroid hormone may have raised the muscle calcium slightly. Dixon *et al.* (1929) also found that parathyroid tetany did not affect the muscle calcium. Haury (1930) found that the calcium content of muscle, calculated on a dry-weight basis, was lowered in rachitic animals. Linder (1940) reported in rats that a rachitogenic diet raised the brain calcium but left the liver calcium unchanged. Acute ergosterol poisoning raised both the liver and brain calcium.

The administration of calcium salts apparently has little effect on the calcium content of tissues. Heubner and Rona (1923) found that injection of $CaCl_2$ into cats in acute experiments increased only the kidney calcium. In chronic experiments the calcium of the heart and liver possibly rose.

Phosphorus Content of the Body

Much less work has been done in this area. Iob and Swanson (1934) found the phosphorus content of human fetuses to rise gradually on a body weight basis from 3 months to term. Widdowson and Spray (1951) reported the same gradual rise, the phosphorus content at term being 0.46%. Economou-Mavrou and McCance (1958) found the fetal serum phosphorus to be about 4 times that of the mother; this is also found in young children. The total muscle phosphorus was about half that of maternal muscle.

The body phosphorus during growth has been determined mainly in animals. Cox and Imboden (1936) reported that the newborn rat was almost uncalcified, but its composition was fairly constant in spite of wide changes in the maternal diet. Sherman and Quinn (1926) found in growing rats that the rate of increase in total phosphorus content rose faster than that of growth but that the total calcium increased at a still faster rate. When calcification was complete about 80% of the total phosphorus was in the skeleton. Animals raised on low phosphorus diets contained less phosphorus during the period of most active growth, but caught up with the controls when growth ceased. Mitchell and his colleagues, in the three papers mentioned above, also reported the phosphorus content of the bodies they analyzed, the figure on a fat-free basis varying between 0.77 and 1.16%. On recalculating the figures of Forbes *et al.* (1956), it was found that about 75% of the total phosphorus was in the skeleton.

The total phosphorus content of various organs has been listed by Katchman (1961), but since the phosphorus is present in so many forms, organic and inorganic, the total figures are somewhat meaningless.

_____ *Chapter 5*

CALCIUM AND PHOSPHORUS
BALANCES AND RETENTION

The classic way of arriving at this information has been the metabolic balance experiment; until labeled isotopes were available, no other method could be used. In essence, an accurate analysis was made of the substance under investigation in the food and in the excreta. By this means it was possible to determine if the subject was in equilibrium, or in positive or negative balance. To obtain accurate results frequently meant the use of a metabolic unit in which the subjects were confined, so that it was not possible for them to eat anything but what was provided, and all the excreta could be collected. In spite of these precautions, many balance experiments, and especially those concerning calcium and phosphorus, gave a fictitiously high level of retention, and it would be suspected that not all the excreta had been collected. Arithmetically, the weakness of the method is that the answer is often a small difference between two large figures and a small error in these large figures can make a substantial difference to the final result.

In addition, the information arrived at only estimated how much of the element being studied went into, or came out, and gave no clue as to its treatment inside the body. As a result of the introduction of the new kinetic methods, using labeled elements, it is now possible to answer

some of these questions. This aspect of calcium and phosphorus metabolism is dealt with in a separate chapter.

Since much of the earlier work has only a historical interest, em-
phasis will be placed on the more recent balance work which seems
to be more accurate. A very good evaluation of balance methods has
been written by Isaksson and Sjögren (1967).

Calcium Loss in Sweat

An important finding is that calcium can be lost in significant
amounts in sweat, especially under hot conditions. Consolazio *et al.*
(1962) reported that as much as 20 mg/hour could be lost in this way;
consequently, with heavy sweating the loss might be 30% of the total
excretion. Urinary calcium did not decrease in compensation for that
lost in the sweat, even in man acclimated to work at high temperatures.
Vellar (1968) found, with forced sweating, that the sweat contained
0.64 mg/10 ml, the loss being 8 mg/hour; Isaksson and Sjögren commented that ignoring these losses could make a substantial change in
the balance picture. However, the loss of phosphorus in sweat was
negligible.

Other dermal losses of calcium or phosphorus in hair (Johnston *et al.*,
1958) or nails (Vellar, 1970) are so small that they can be disregarded.

Adaptation to Low Calcium Intakes

Another important phenomenon is the ability to adapt to low
calcium intakes. This has been demonstrated in children and adults as
well as in rats, and the literature up to 1944 has been summarized by
Mitchell (1944). This ability to adapt has made it almost impossible to
arrive at a figure for daily calcium requirements. Thus Hegsted *et al.*
(1952) found persons in Lima, Peru, in equilibrium on intakes as low as
100–200 mg/day. Nicolaysen *et al.* (1953) reported that 13 of their 14
male subjects adapted to low calcium intakes in from 2 to 8 months.

Several people have found that calcium retention depends on the
previous calcium intake. Walker *et al.* (1948) put subjects on to a low
calcium diet after they had been subsisting at a high calcium level. They
all went into negative calcium balance, which became less negative

with time, and finally the subjects went into equilibrium. Johnston *et al.* (1956) reported that the higher the previous calcium intake, the greater the calcium loss on the lower intake. Rottensten as long ago as 1938 suggested that the mechanism of adjustment was a function of the calcium stores in the body; as they became depleted, the calcium requirement was reduced.

Calcium and Phosphorus Studies

IN INFANTS

A number of balance studies have been done on infants, both breast-fed and on formulas. Slater (1961) investigated normal full-term baby boys on the sixth, seventh, and eight day of age. The average intake of calcium and phosphorus, stated on a mg/kg/day basis, were 36 and 20, respectively, in babies on human milk, and 135 and 103, respectively, in bottle-fed babies. The percentage retention of calcium was higher with the formula babies, but the retention of phosphorus was almost twice as high in the breast-fed babies compared to those bottle-fed. The bottle-fed babies lost much calcium in the feces. He considered, since the bottle-fed babies lost much less calcium in the urine, that the low phosphorus content of human milk could be a limiting factor in the retention of calcium (and also magnesium). Incidentally, the phosphorus content of the urine of the breast-fed babies was almost zero. Lough *et al.* (1963) studied slightly older babies, 25 to 46 days of age, which were bottle-fed. The calcium intake averaged 140 mg/kg/day and the retention was around 42 mg/kg/day. Similar figures for calcium were reported by Harrison *et al.* (1955) and for calcium and phosphorus by Williams *et al.* (1970). The figures for calcium are interesting, since it is usually held that 10 mg/kg/day is adequate for adults.

Widdowson *et al.* (1963) came to the same conclusion as Slater, namely, that the phosphorus in the milk of breast-fed babies might be a limiting factor in calcium retention. They studied babies from the fifth to the eighth day of life and found that phosphorus added to breast milk increased calcium absorption and reduced that in the urine; they concluded that calcification of bone and soft tissue growth at this age period were enhanced by giving more phosphorus.

It is of interest, as pointed out by Bunge (1898), that the calcium content of the milk has a relationship with the rate of growth of the young, as the figures in the following tabulation show.

Species	Days to double birth weight	% Ca in mother's milk
Man	180	0.02
Cow	47	0.12
Dog	7	0.32

Davies *et al.* (1964) reported that young rabbits doubled their birth weight by about the sixth day, the calcium in the milk being 517, and the phosphorus 274 mg/100 g.

IN CHILDREN

The calcium and phosphorus intakes of children have been reported by a number of workers. Most of the investigations, in which the children were on normal diets, show an increase in calcium and phosphorus intake with age (Beal, 1954). Burke *et al.* (1962) carried out a longitudinal study on boys and girls from 1 to 18 years of age, all being healthy and on normal diets. From 1 to 2 years old, boys consumed on an average 0.89 g Ca/day; girls, 0.91 g Ca. The boys' intake rose to a maximum at 18 years, 1.68 g/day, but girls reached a maximum between 15 and 18 years of 1.20 g/day, and by the time they reached 18 were getting 1.08 g/day. It is a pity that these results were not stated on a weight basis, as there was considerable variation when stated in absolute amounts. It is of interest to compare these findings with the older ones of Mitchell *et al.* (1945) or Irving (1950b). These writers tried to work out the requirement of calcium based on what was then known of the daily increments of calcium into the body. In both cases the figures arrived at were much lower than those of Beal or Burke *et al.*

Children in underdeveloped countries can apparently "get along" on calcium intakes far lower than those in the United States. Kantha *et al.* (1957) reported on undernourished children aged 8–11 years who were habitually on a poor vegetarian diet or one that was supplemented with vitamins, calcium, and phosphorus. Average figures were as follows: The calcium intake on the poor diet was 287 mg/day and the supplemented diet gave 565 mg daily. The retentions were respectively 53 and 194 mg, on both levels the children being in positive calcium balance. The basal phosphorus intake was 421 mg/day and the supplemented one, 796 mg, and the retentions were respectively 76 mg and 164 mg/day. Begum and Pereira (1969) similarly investigated children aged 3–5 years who had been on a calcium intake of about 200 mg/day for several months. They were all in positive balance and had a retention of about 38.5%. The retention was increased by giving more calcium, indicating that their stores were not filled; interestingly enough, giving lysine supplements had no effect upon the retention. Flores and Garcia (1960) have also reported that although the calcium intake of preschool children in Guatemala was very low, the children did not have rickets.

In Adults

Schofield et al. (1956) and Scoular et al. (1957) gave figures for calcium and phosphorus balances in young college women. The latter study showed that with self-selected diets, the calcium intake could be as high as 1.7 g/day and the phosphorus over 1 g. Brieter et al. (1941) many years ago found that there were high and low calcium utilizers, and Nicolaysen et al. (1953) more recently reported that individuals on a constant calcium intake and observed over long periods of time abruptly changed their retentions and went for no apparent reason from positive to negative balance, and back again, the changes being caused chiefly by alterations in fecal excretion.

The mutual effects of calcium and phosphorus upon their respective retentions have also been investigated. It was stated above that possibly the phosphorus content of the diet of babies could influence calcium retention. Johnston and Folsom (1961) reported a converse finding in adults, in that while they could be in calcium equilibrium on low intakes, they might be in negative phosphorus balance on intakes generally considered adequate. This could be rectified by increasing the calcium intake.

While high levels of phosphate in the diet depress calcium retention in animals, it is unlikely that such effect occur in man on diets usually eaten. Human dietaries almost without exception contain much more phosphorus than calcium, but this imbalance does not affect calcium metabolism. Studies have shown that the ingestion of large amounts of phosphorus as phosphate or as H_3PO_4 have within wide limits no effect upon the calcium balance. Malm (1953) gave adult men phosphoric acid at levels from 0.8 to 3.16 g (250–1000 mg P) daily for several weeks. The calcium intake varied from 450 to 950 mg/day. No effect at all was seen on the calcium balance.

The same was found when the phosphorus was given as a neutral Na–K mixture to increase the level of intake of phosphorus from 1.4 to 2.0 g daily, the calcium intake being 0.5 g/day. H. Lauersen (private communication, 1948) tested the effects of the daily ingestion of 5 g of $NaH_2PO_4 \cdot 2H_2O$ or 2 g of H_3PO_4 on human adults. In both cases no effect upon calcium excretion was noted. Baylor et al. (1950) found the same with a woman who was given 2000 mg phosphorus as phosphate daily. Nicolaysen et al. (1953) quote from their extensive unpublished material which supports the findings of Malm.

Spencer et al. (1965) conducted experiments with different levels of calcium and phosphorus intake and found that the level of calcium in the diet did not affect phosphorus balance, when the calcium content of the diet gave 200 or 1500 mg/day, the phosphorus content of the diet giving 500 or 1700 mg/day. However, increasing the phosphorus intake did improve slightly the calcium balance on both levels of intake. It may be concluded on the balance of the evidence that quite large increases in phosphorus ingestion, either as phosphoric acid or neutral phosphate, do not affect calcium metabolism in man to any significant extent.

In an effort to avoid balance experiments, D. E. Williams et al. (1964) suggested measuring bone density to evaluate the calcium status. They claimed that this measurement correlated well with the calcium content of the diet.

During Space Flight

It has long been known that continuous bed rest can affect the metabolism of several elements. Issekutz et al. (1966) found that bed rest caused a marked increase in urinary calcium excretion which was not prevented by a high calcium intake or exercise while lying down. They concluded that the calcium loss was due to a prolonged absence of longitudinal pressure on the bones, rather than physical inactivity. These findings had a practical application in studies of the calcium metabolism of astronauts during space flights.

Mack and LaChance (1967) X-rayed the os calcis for bone density and reported that there was a loss of density following the Gemini V mission, when the austronauts were on a low calcium intake; this loss was less during the Gemini IV flight when the calcium intake was higher, and least on the Gemini VII mission, when the two crew members had intakes of 945 and 921 mg/day, respectively. The authors considered the calcium intake more significant than the length of the flight, as Gemini VII had the longest duration. They also thought that isometric and isotonic exercises, which could be performed during the mission, were of importance.

Hegsted (1967) criticized these findings, as he doubted the value of bone density measurements. The variations in these measurements taken on the ground before and after the flight were as great as those during the space flight. Reid *et al.* (1968) arranged for the collection of excreta and other data for balance experiments on several elements, including calcium and phosphorus, during the Gemini VII flight. The difficulties in carrying these procedures out during the mission were great. They reported that the astronauts were in calcium equilibrium, and slightly negative nitrogen and phosphorus balance, presumably due to loss of muscle mass. However in view of the fact that even under optimal conditions, balance experiments tend to fictitious positive balances, and that conditions during the flight were certainly not optimal, results of Reid *et al.* must be accepted with reserve. No doubt other investigations will show if these findings were correct.

DURING PREGNANCY

Little recent work has been done on calcium and phosphorus metabolism during pregnancy and lactation. From the point of view of calcium metabolism, pregnancy has but a slight effect on the healthy organism. In the case of the human, calcification of the fetus demands 35 g of calcium at the very most, which means a drain of about 3.5%

from the maternal stores, presuming that no supplemental calcium was given in the diet. In the case of the rat, rabbit, and mouse (Spray and Widdowson, 1950), the newborn animal is virtually calcium-free and its calcification imposes little strain on the mother.

The first and classic balance investigation was carried out by Hoff-ström (1910), who studied a woman from the seventeenth week to term. The calcium balance was positive most of the time, just enough calcium being stored for the needs of the fetus. Many workers have reported, on the other hand, that at the end of gestation the maternal organism has stored far more calcium than needed for the products of conception. Thus Goss and Schmidt (1930) found that during preg-nancy rats stored 4–5 times as much calcium as was contained in the fetus, placenta, and uterus. Even if the young were resorbed owing to vitamin E deficiency, this extra storage of calcium still occurred. Forbes et al. (1922) found a rapid storage of calcium at the end of gestation in cows and Landsberg (1915) has reported the same for women. Coons and Coons (1935) studied a case from weeks 31 to 35 of pregnancy and found calcium storage at a lower level. Thus there appears to be considerable variation in the storage of calcium at the end of pregnancy; since the previous calcium intake has not always been considered, it is quite possible that this may have been insufficient, especially as the calcium intake is often deliberately increased during pregnancy. It seems safe to conclude that any extra storage of calcium in the mother's body during pregnancy is due to previous deficiency, and if the calcium intake has been adequate, calcium storage does not occur.

This is especially seen in cases reported by Shenolikar (1970) of pregnant women on calcium intakes of 400 mg/day. They were in negative calcium balance during the first trimester, but went into pos-itive balance in the second and third trimesters.

The calcium intake is, however, important for the fertility and health of the mother, apart from the calcium requirement of the fetus. Thus rats on a low calcium intake were either infertile or ate their young, or the young died in utero (Toverud 1923–1924; Macomber, 1927). Davidson (1930) found with pigs that a low calcium diet greatly in-creased the number of piglets born dead. This is probably not a specific calcium effect, since any type of inadequate diet would presumably interfere with fertility and pregnancy.

DURING LACTATION

From the point of view of calcium metabolism, this imposes a severe strain on the mother. Most experimenters with rats have found them consistently in negative calcium balance. Sherman and Quinn (1926) found that calcium and phosphorus were lost together in lactation and subsequently regained in the same ratio, suggesting that they were both mobilized from bone. Direct analysis by Warnock and Duckworth (1944) showed that the "ends" and cancellous parts of the bones contributed this calcium, the shafts being unaffected. Goss and Schmidt (1930) found that the largest litters caused the greatest losses, as much as 20% of the body calcium being removed from the mother rat. They noted that while the animals appeared to get enough calcium in their diet, they were unable to absorb it fast enough. Kletzien *et al.* (1932) found that with a diet containing 0.67% Ca, the blood calcium was lowered; they suggested that mobilization was unable to keep up with the demands of the mammary glands. Bronner (1960) found in rats that about 10–15% of the milk or filial calcium was maternal in origin.

Cows can apparently be kept in calcium equilibrium during lactation if the intake is enough (Hart *et al.*, 1926–1927; Huffman *et al.*, 1930), but as a rule, even with apparently adequate supplies, they are in negative calcium balance (Hart *et al.*, 1922; Turner and Hartman, 1928–1929). Both Forbes *et al.* (1922) and Huffman *et al.* found that cows which were in negative calcium balance early in lactation, or during the height of lactation, could make this up afterward by retaining calcium again. Forbes *et al.* considered that the calcium of the bones was more available for milk formation than that of the diet and doubted whether supplementary calcium in the diet was used at all for lactation purposes, though Huffman *et al.* showed that calcium utilization was more efficient during heavy milking.

Work on lactating women has shown that these findings also apply to them. Hunscher (1930) investigated three lactating women and found that in spite of large intakes the negativity of the calcium balance increased after 6 months of high milk production, the calcium being lost mainly in the feces, and in fact to such an extent that the fecal loss sometimes exceeded the whole intake. Here, too, the bone calcium was presumably more available than the food calcium. In late lactation, when less milk was secreted, calcium was again stored in the body.

Donelson *et al.* (1931) and Hummel *et al.* (1936) reported negative balances during lactation; but if the calcium intake is adequate, calcium can be retained (Oberst and Plass, 1940), the retention being lowest with the greatest milk production. In this report the calcium intakes were from 1.92 to 2.18 g per day. Shukers *et al.* (1931) found that lactating, women, allowed to choose their own food, increased their calcium intake 62–88% over that during pregnancy, the daily intakes being from 2.03 to 5.3 g, far higher than usually taken.

These facts illustrate the remarkable elasticity of the body in dealing with emergencies in calcium metabolism. During periods of calcium demand, large amounts can be given up to be regained again when the need falls. Whether it is physiological for such large losses to be sustained in another question. It must happen in the majority of cases that provided the stores are well filled at the end of pregnancy, and provided further that they will be replenished after lactation has ended, no harm ensues. In the case of women starting off with low reserves, on the other hand, it is obvious that serious results may ensue, as they will probably have little opportunity of refilling their stores, especially if subsequent pregnancies follow rapidly.

While these problems are probably of only academic interest in Western countries, whose populations are well or overfed, and where nutritional factors during pregnancy and lactation are taken care of at special clinics, they are of paramount importance in underdeveloped countries, where they may cause considerable maternal morbidity.

_____ *Chapter 6*

RECOMMENDED DAILY CALCIUM AND PHOSPHORUS REQUIREMENTS

Calcium Requirements

In Adults

The current recommended daily requirements are based on the older papers of Leitch (1936–1937) and Mitchell and Curzon (1939). Since at that time a good deal of thought was given to this question, it is of interest to follow the methods they used. Leitch selected from the literature a large number of balance data on healthy women both in positive and negative balance. On plotting intake against output, the level of calcium intake above which losses and gains of calcium were equal was 550 mg/day. This worked out at almost 10 mg/kg body weight. Mitchell and Curzon selected 139 observations from the literature on 107 subjects, of whom 18 were men. These results were plotted with respect to intake and output and a straight line fitted to the data. This line intersected the diagonal at 9.75 mg/kg body weight/day, a figure that agrees well with that of Leitch obtained by an analogous method.

In a study of 9 normal male subjects (Steggerda and Mitchell, 1941) when the availability of milk calcium was being investigated, an average calcium requirement of 9.55 mg/kg body weight/day was arrived at. In 1946 Steggerda and Mitchell did balance experiments on 19 men, the diet periods being 20 days and 75 such periods being considered. Averaging all the results, the daily calcium requirement came to 9.21 mg/kg body weight. In a later paper from the same laboratory Bricker *et al.* (1949), working with 8 women, found that the requirement was 11.8 mg/kg body weight/day.

In their 1946 paper, Steggerda and Mitchell summarized their present and earlier findings, certain unpublished data, and also calculations from the work of Breiter *et al.* (1941), who conducted similar balance experiments. The mean of the daily calcium requirement per kilogram of body weight varied from 9.21 to 11.61 mg, and averaged 9.99 mg for 43 individuals.

They recommended an intake of 10 mg/kg body weight/day, provided that an average proportion of calcium came from dairy products. They did not feel that a "margin of safety" was needed. In the

TABLE I

DAILY ALLOWANCES OF CALCIUM AND PHOSPHORUS RECOMMENDED BY THE FOOD AND NUTRITION BOARD OF THE NATIONAL ACADEMY OF SCIENCES – NATIONAL RESEARCH COUNCIL

Subjects	Age	Calcium (g)	Phosphorus (g)
Both sexes	$0-\frac{1}{6}$	0.4	0.2
	$\frac{1}{6}-\frac{1}{2}$	0.5	0.4
	$\frac{1}{2}-1$	0.6	0.5
	1–2	0.7	0.7
	2–6	0.8	0.8
	6–8	0.9	0.9
	8–10	1.0	1.0
Males	10–12	1.2	1.2
	12–18	1.4	1.4
	18–75+	0.8	0.8
Females	10–12	1.2	1.2
	12–18	1.3	1.3
	18–75+	0.8	0.8
Pregnancy		+0.4	+0.4
Lactation		+0.5	+0.5

case of the individual who had been accustomed to more, the adaptive mechanism would take effect and, judging from the experiments quoted elsewhere, would cause no physiological disturbance at this level of intake.

The National Academy of Sciences and the National Research Council in their publication "Recommended Dietary Allowances" (1968) have suggested a daily intake of 0.8 g for both sexes (see Table I).

IN INFANTS

Based on the figures given in the section of calcium balances in infants, the figure of 0.4–0.6 g Ca/day, suggested by the Academy and Council, during the first 12 months of life, appears to be adequate, but the source of the calcium is an important factor.

IN CHILDREN

The figures given follow fairly closely those reported from balance experiments (e.g., Burke *et al.*, 1962) and are certainly adequate. They are, however, far higher than those calculated by Mitchell *et al.* (1945) or Irving (1950b) from known daily calcium increments in the body.

DURING PREGNANCY

Since the products of conception at term contain at most only about 25 g of calcium, very little extra calcium need be given to supply this amount. However, as a margin of safety, 400 mg of extra calcium per day is recommended.

DURING LACTATION

As pointed out elsewhere, this process can be a considerable drain on the mother's calcium reserves and, in spite of large supplements in the diet, it has been reported that both cows and humans may be in negative balance. Left to themselves, women many take large amounts of extra calcium. The recommended allowance of 500 mg extra calcium daily is probably not adequate for a woman in high lactation, but is a considerable help in offsetting the drain on her reserves.

The recommendations of official bodies of other countries are on the whole similar to those of the United States. The allowances for children in Great Britain are higher, while the allowances for adults suggested by FAO (Food and Agriculture Organization, 1962) are considerably lower (0.4–0.5 g/day).

Phosphorus

The requirements for phosphorus follow closely those for calcium.

_____ *Chapter 7*

BLOOD CALCIUM AND PHOSPHORUS

Blood Calcium

The blood calcium of man is remarkably constant and its regulation is significantly affected by the parathyroid gland, as described elsewhere. The cation is almost entirely in the plasma at a level varying from 2.3 to 2.5 mM. Keating *et al.* (1969) examined over 500 normal human subjects of both sexes, over a wide range of ages. In man the value at 20 years was on an average of 2.4 mM and fell slightly with age, while in women the value of 2.4 mM was constant over the age period studied, up to 80 years. This constancy is seen in many other animals, but in the rabbit the plasma level is subject to great variations, rising as high as 7.75 mM under normal conditions.

Although it is usually stated that the red blood cells contain no calcium, human red cells were found to be associated with calcium at a level of 0.63 μg/ml of packed cell volume as determined by atomic absorption spectrophotometry (Harrison and Long, 1968). This calcium is associated with the cell membrane and remains in the ghost cells after osmotic hemolysis, in contrast to magnesium and zinc. EDTA removed 90% of this calcium without hemolysis. Long and

Mouat (1971) reported that the calcium binding sites on the red cell membrane were mostly ionized carboxyl groups of sialic acid residues and N-acetylneuraminic acid. Most recently Romero and Whittam (1971) suggested that the calcium content of the red cell was kept low by a calcium pump that utilized ATP for energy.

Forms of Blood Calcium

DIFFUSIBLE

It had long been known that calcium was present in a diffusible and nondiffusible form, but the determination presented some difficulties. The earlier investigators had to use indirect methods. Thus if simple dialysis is carried out, all the calcium will be removed from serum, since the two fractions are in equilibrium. Instead, a procedure known as compensation dialysis can be used, in which serum is dialyzed against a number of solutions of different calcium content. The solution in which no change of calcium concentration occurs contains calcium ions at the same level as the serum. With this method, about 60% of human serum is found to be diffusible. Greene and Power (1931), using the method of vividiffusion, in which the entire blood of a living animal is dialyzed against a small volume of fluid, reported on an average 62% of the calcium to be diffusible. Ultrafiltration under pressure through a collodion membrane gives figures of much the same order (Greenberg and Larson, 1935). McLean and Hastings (1935a) made use of the sensitivity of the frog heart to calcium ions and found about half the total serum calcium to be diffusible and nearly all of this in an ionized state. Calculations based on the composition of cerebrospinal fluid, edema fluid, ascites or pleural effusions indicate that the diffusible calcium of normal serum is about 1.25 mM.

Subsequent work using different methods has in general confirmed these findings. Thus Ettori and Scoggan (1959), using a method based on the absorbance of metal indicators at two wavelengths, found the ionized calcium to be about 1.3 mM. Chutkow (1968), using atomic absorption spectrophotometry, reported the ionized calcium to be 1.7 mM. Moore (1970) employed ion-exchange electrodes to determine the ionic calcium directly and obtained values of 0.94–1.33 mM, but this method is known to have many technical difficulties.

Walser (1961c) has calculated the various fractions of calcium in human plasma. He estimated the amounts of various ion species in plasma ultrafiltrate. The proportion of each bound to protein was estimated by applying appropriate corrections for the Donnan factor and for plasma water content. The determination of free cation concentrations together with the revelant stability constants permitted calculation of the concentration of each complex in a mixed electrolyte solution from these values, plus total measured concentrations of individual anionic ligands. The calcium figures he reported are shown in the following tabulation.

Calcium fraction	Percent
Free ions	47.5
Protein bound	46.0
$CaHPO_4$	1.6
Calcium citrate	1.7
Unidentified complexes	3.2

NONDIFFUSIBLE

Turning to the nature of the nondiffusible fraction, there seems hardly any need to consider the older views, since all evidence now points to this being a calcium–protein complex. McLean and Hastings (1935a) showed beyond doubt that a relationship exists between the calcium ions and the protein in plasma; they have calculated mass-action equations and ionization constants. They have constructed a nomogram from which, knowing the values of total protein and total calcium, the calcium ion concentration can be derived. The mass-action considerations involved have been shown to be true, as regards the proportion of ionized and un-ionized calcium, over a wide range of values as in hypo-and hyperparathyroidism, provided the protein content of the plasma does not change.

The ability of blood protein to bind calcium has been demonstrated by a number of workers. McLean and Hastings (1935b) first attempted a quantitative study with purified albumins prepared from the sera of horses and oxen. Martin and Perkins (1950) found the serum albumin of horse and ox to bind about II mg/g nitrogen: in humans the corresponding figure was 4.7–4.8 mg. Repeated recrystallization could alter this binding power. In a subsequent paper (1953) the binding power of human albumin was found to be very constant at 4.7 mg ±0.9 mg/g nitrogen from ages 2 to 91, and the same in both sexes.

Carr (1953) reported that bovine albumin took up a maximum number of 8 calcium ions per molecule of protein at a pH of 7. With increased pH the binding power rose, and fell with decreased pH. Loken et al. (1960) reported that calcium was bound in the proportion of 0.10 mM/g protein. The pK of calcium proteinate at pH 7.35 and 35° was 2.18, the same as had been found by McLean and Hastings. Irons and Perkins (1962) compared the binding affinity of calcium, magnesium, and strontium ions to albumin, and found that calcium had the highest affinity, and that the binding was by electrostatic attraction mainly to nonspecific sites. In the presence of citrate the calcium was still bound as the free ion at pH values above 5.2, but below this value it was bound as a negatively charged calcium citrate complex.

As stated above, all calcium can be dialyzed out of serum. Armstrong et al. (1952) investigated this in vivo using ^{45}Ca, and reported that protein binding did not impede the transcapillary movement of calcium and that the redistribution of calcium between the ionized and bound forms was rapid. The transcapillary movement of ^{45}Ca and ^{22}Na were the same. Giese and Comar (1964) found that after giving radioactive calcium to starved sheep, the specific activity of plasma and urine differed, suggesting that there were two forms of calcium in plasma between which calcium would not exchange, one more readily excreted than the other. The two forms were apparently not protein-bound, nor were they dialyzable; under these circumstances some other calcium complex must exist.

The effects of acidosis and alkalosis on the blood calcium have been reported, but the results are contradictory. It would appear that in acidosis a nonultrafiltrable calcium–phosphate complex is formed, but the mechanism underlying it is obscure (Brown and Prasad, 1957; Schaefer et al., 1961). It is well known that phosphate infusions will result in the formation of a colloidal calcium–phosphate complex in the blood (McLean and Hinrichs, 1938) and more recently

Hebert *et al.* (1966) studied this phenomenon further. Phosphate infusions lowered the serum calcium without any loss of calcium from the body. The *in vivo* solubility product of $CaPHO_4$ appeared to be 2.4×10^{-6} moles/liter, which agreed with many previous determinations *in vitro*, and the serum calcium fell in direct proportion as the solubility product was exceeded during phosphate infusion.

The mobilization of calcium for the blood has been studied by Symonds and Treacher (1968). They put the circulation of goats in series with cation exchange columns and only calcium was affected. Forty percent of the calcium was removed in 30 minutes and normal values were regained within 2 hours of terminating calcium removal. Mobilization reached a maximum 15–20 minutes after calcium removal began and then declined rapidly. According to Bronner and Aubert (1965) bone resorption is the chief regulator of the plasma calcium level and this process presumably acted during the calcium depletion experiments.

Blood Calcium and Egg-Laying

Another aspect, the blood changes in hens during the egg-laying period, has been studied. At this time both the total (Riddle and Reinhart, 1926) and nondiffusible calcium in the plasma rise (Correll and Hughes, 1933). Clegg and Hein (1953) found that after giving diethylstilboesterol the rise in nondiffusible calcium in chick serum was paralleled by a rise in concentration of two of the electrophoretic components; in a later paper, Ericson *et al.* (1955) after similar treatment found a "new" protein that was rich in phosphorus and identified with ^{32}P. When the calcium in the serum was raised, the electrophoretic mobility of this protein was markedly reduced, but that of the others was not, and this was attributed to combination with calcium. The nature of the new proteins in plasma has been investigated by Schjeide and Urist (1956, 1959). They injected estrone into roosters and found at least two new protein components which they called X1 and X2. The raised serum calcium was associated with X1, which was a phosphoprotein and has subsequently been shown to be phosvitin (Benowitz and Terepka, 1968). Both these latter authors and also Schjeide and Urist stated that the raised nondiffusible calcium after estrogen injections was due solely to complexing with compound X1 or phosvitin in blood, there being no change in the ionized or ultrafiltrable components. Benowitz and Terepka found phosvitin to bind calcium on a molar Ca:P basis of about 1:1, multiple serine phosphates complexing calcium directly. Schjeide and Urist (1959) reported that X2 component was a lipoprotein and did not bind calcium to any appreciable extent. Hurwitz (1968) found in laying hens that the total calcium rose to over 7 mM, of which 5.5 mM was rapidly exchangeable and 1.6 mM slowly exchangeable. Urist *et al.* (1960) postulated that under these conditions parathyroid hormone controlled ultrafiltrable calcium and estrogen the nonultrafiltrable, by causing the formation of a phosphoprotein in the liver which complexed calcium.

Other species have been investigated and similar changes found. Thus Dessauer *et al.* (1956) reported a large increase in blood calcium, magnesium, and total protein during estrus in viviparous colubrid snakes. *Xenopus laevis* formed a new calcium-binding serum protein after injection of estrogen (Munday *et al.*, 1968) and Urist and Schjeide (1961) reported that all vertebrates except elasmobranchs and mammals had hypercalcemia and hyperproteinemia after estrogen injections. Teleosts, amphibia, and reptiles produced a new component very like the X2 fraction they had found in birds. But estrogens, although causing medullary bone formation in mice, have no effect upon their blood levels of calcium or phosphorus.

None of these other species produce eggs with calcified shells. Furthermore, Schjeide and Urist (1959) found both the X1 and X2 proteins in chick egg yolk. It may therefore be asked whether these proteins, which are synthesized in the liver, are not primarily intended to be deposited in egg yolk, and that the ability of one to complex with calcium was a lucky break for birds!

Blood Phosphorus

Phosphorus is present in whole blood in at least two forms, esters and phosphate ions, and possibly a third, a bound form, as will be discussed later. The esters are in the cellular elements (Kay, 1928), are of metabolic importance, and will not be considered further here, except to say that they are readily hydrolyzed in shed blood if it is allowed to stand, so that inorganic phosphate must be quickly estimated, or the responsible enzymes inactivated.

Phosphate ions are present in the plasma and are usually expressed as phosphorus, which is at a level of 1–2 mM in adults. Keating *et al.* (1969) reported on over 500 subjects of both sexes and found that in men the average value fell from about 1.13 mM at age 20 to about 0.97 mM at 80. The values in women were similar, fell slightly from ages 20 to 30 and then rose slightly with age up to 80. Babies have a consistently higher phosphorus level. Pigs have a level of about 2.6 mM and sheep, oxen, and goats likewise have values higher than humans (Kay, 1928).

Homeostasis of Plasma Phosphate

This is still not completely understood. The phosphorus level in blood is not nearly so constant as is that of calcium. This is not difficult to understand since the blood phosphorus is in equilibrium not only with bone phosphorus, but with that arising from a large number of organic phosphorus compounds produced as a result of cellular metabolism. The hyperphosphatemia of infants has been attributed to the influence of growth hormone (Reifenstein *et al.*, 1946), since patients with active adenomas of the hypophysis tend to have higher blood phosphorus levels.

Probably the major control is through the kidney. Howard (1954) reported that patients with renal insufficiency had raised serum phosphorus levels, and while feeding excess amounts of calcium, aluminum, or iron to normal people had no effect on the blood phosphorus, these elements caused an abrupt fall in serum phosphorus in patients with renal insufficiency. As pointed out elsewhere, the parathyroid gland regulates renal phosphorus excretion. Although parathyroid hormone caused only a small effect on phosphorus excretion in normal subjects (Handler *et al.*, 1951), it produced a large phosphorus diuresis in hypoparathyroid patients (Ellsworth and Howard, 1934).

Howard (1954) thought that cellular phosphorus more than bone phosphorus was concerned in phosphorus homeostasis. More recent work confirms this view. Symonds and Treacher (1967) perfused the circulation of goats through anion exchange columns, inorganic phosphate being selectively removed. A fall of up to 50% in blood phosphorus occurred in 30 minutes. The mobilization of phosphorus was very rapid at first, and then fell off, suggesting an initial store that had been depleted. The phosphorus level returned to normal within 80 minutes of stopping the perfusion. The mobilized phosphorus did not come from saliva, organic phosphorus compounds in the blood, or bone, but presumably from cellular phosphorus. Thus a mechanism existed which responded to small changes in plasma phosphorus, but could not be very effective, as plasma phosphorus undergoes spontaneous wide variations. Many years ago Gaunt et al. (1942) reported that animals depleted of calcium and phosphorus stored more ^{32}P in their muscles than did nondepleted animals, suggesting that muscle could act as a phosphorus store. Schneider and Steenbock (1939) had found that under certain conditions the soft tissues could yield phosphorus for use in other parts of the body. As stated elsewhere, parathyroid hormone has been postulated to control calcium and phosphorus movement between extra- and intracellular fluid and also to have an intracellular action. It is thus possible that in addition to its action on phosphate excretion, the parathyroid gland regulates phosphorus mobilization from soft tissues in its control of phosphorus homeostasis.

Forms of Phosphorus in the Blood

Phosphorus is present as the ions of orthophosphoric acid and Levinskas (1953) has considered the ionization of orthophosphate at the ionic strength and pH of plasma. He calculated that the proportional concentration of the $H_2PO_4^-$ ion was 18.65%, that of HPO_4^{2-} was 81.4%, and that of the PO_3^{3-} ion was 8×10^{-3}%. The respective activities were 0.12×10^{-3}, 0.19×10^{-3}, and 5×10^{-6}. Since by definition calcium and phosphorus in plasma and extracellular fluid are in equilibrium with the exchangeable phase of the bone mineral, it should be possible to select an activity product showing the least variation in describing the solubility of this salt. Levinskas found that the expression, $aCa^{2+} \cdot aHPO_4^{2-}$ filled these requirements best.

McLean et al. (1964) had drawn curves of the solubility product constants of $CaHPO_4$ and of $Ca_3(PO_4)_2$ as related to pH and phosphorus content of the solution. They superimposed the minimum ion concentrations at which calcification of hypertrophic cartilage occurred *in vitro*, and found that at pH's above 7.3 calcification was correlated with the solubility product of $CaHPO_4$, whose ion product seemed to be the determining factor in the process, which corresponds well with Levinskas's calculations.

Nonultrafiltrable Phosphorus

The question of the existence of a nonultrafiltrable fraction of phosphorus in the blood has been frequently discussed. There is abundant evidence that under experimental conditions a colloidal calcium–phosphorus complex can be formed. If animals with low phosphorus rickets are starved, the blood phosphorus rises owing to mobilization from the soft tissues, and the calcium falls, often to tetanic levels (Irving and Nienaber, 1946). McLean and Hinrichs (1938) found that injected phosphorus formed a colloidal complex with calcium which was rapidly removed from the blood.

Grollman (1927) first reported all the inorganic phosphorus in the plasma of the dog and pig to be ultrafiltrable, as was confirmed by Hogben and Bollman (1951) and others. Further studies cast doubt upon this conclusion, especially those in which the specific activities of plasma and urine were compared after injection of ^{32}P, the specific activity of urine being much higher than that of the blood. Govaerts (1952) considered that there was a "mineral" form of phosphorus which was easily excreted and another form not excretable and different from the mineral form. Fuchs and Fuchs (1954) confirmed these findings and reported that if a donor animal was injected with ^{32}P and then 1 hour later its plasma was transfused into another animal, the specific activity of urine and plasma were identical. They thought that 10% of the blood phosphorus was in a labile, nondiffusible form, which was changed into inorganic phosphorus during chemical estimation.

Some authors, while confirming the above findings, had another explanation—that there was a time lag between the time that phosphorus was filtered through the glomerulus of the kidney and when it reached the bladder (Handler and Cohn, 1951) or that a considerable time had to elapse before equilibrium between plasma and urine occurred (Liljestrand and Swedin, 1952). When this interval was taken into account, the specific activity of plasma and urine was the same.

However, there is convincing evidence that plasma phosphorus is in part bound to protein. Walser (1960, 1961c) used arguments very similar to those reported above for calcium. He estimated the phosphorus in plasma ultrafiltrates and compared this value with that in plasma itself. From the water content of plasma (930 g/liter) and the appropriate Donnan factor for plasma phosphate, he concluded that 12% of plasma phosphorus was bound to protein. Loken et al. (1960) also reported that phosphate was significantly bound to plasma proteins. It thus seems likely on the balance of the evidence that phosphorus is bound in a manner analogous to calcium, but that the linkage is probably more labile than in the case of calcium, and is probably due to physicochemical conditions in plasma.

Endocrine Factors and the Blood Calcium and Phosphorus Levels

The influence of parathyroid hormone, and calcitonin and estrogen are discussed elsewhere. Insulin very probably increases the blood calcium, but secondarily to its effect of lowering the inorganic phosphorus level. The thyroid has a considerable effect upon calcium excretion and in thyrotoxicosis there is an increased loss of calcium. There seems to be no unanimity about the level of blood calcium in this condition. Albright et al. (1931) considered it to be slightly raised, but Wade (1929) found it to be lowered. Robertson (1941) reported that it was lowered from an average figure of 2.6–2.4 mM, the difference proving to be statistically significant. In myxoedema the level is unchanged.

Cortisone causes a greatly increased excretion of calcium in the urine and feces, but in otherwise normal animals both cortisone and adrenocorticotropic hormone cause little change in the blood calcium or, if anything, a fall (Pincus et al., 1951). If, however, the animal is nephrectomized, cortisone causes an increase of serum calcium to toxic levels (Grollman, 1954). Adrenalin administration is followed by a rise in serum calcium (Pincus et al. (1951).

Reports in the literature concerning the hypophysis are somewhat conflicting. Anderson and Oastler (1938), in well-controlled experiments with rats, found that hypophysectomy had no effect upon the blood calcium level, and assumed that the existence of a parathyrotropic hormone in the hypophysis was not proved, which is still the consensus of opinion.

Dietary Factors and the Blood Calcium and Phosphorus Levels

Essentially the chief constituents of the diet that significantly affect these levels are calcium, phosphorus, and vitamin D. The latter is dealt with elsewhere. Twenty-four weeks of semistarvation had no effect on the plasma phosphorus of humans (Keys *et al.*, 1950). The same has been found within limits in rats, but calcium deficiency will in the end cause the blood calcium to fall. Greenberg and Miller (1941) found that a calcium-deficient diet fed to growing rats caused a fall in the blood figure from an original level of 2.5–3.1 mM to one of 1.8 mM after 40 days and to 1.5 mM at 68 days. By this time the body calcium stores had fallen to less than half and the authors considered that a significant reduction in the calcium stores must take place before the blood calcium is reduced.

In animals with well-marked low phosphorus rickets, as caused by the Steenbock–Black diet, the blood calcium level is usually a high normal and the blood inorganic phosphorus greatly lowered. When animals on a low calcium diet are starved, the blood calcium remains at a constant low level for as long as 10 days (Irving, 1946) and presumably is kept depressed by the continual mobilization of phosphate. A rapid and fatal hypocalcemia can be induced by the injection of ethylenediaminetetracetic acid (Popocivi *et al.*, 1950).

Chapter 8

BONE FORMATION AND RESORPTION

Bone Formation

There is a close correlation between the structure of bone, especially during development, and its chemical changes, and a brief account of the microscopic appearances will be given. Furthermore, certain parts of the bone, especially the rachitic growth plate, have been used in enzyme studies. The reader who wants a more complete description is referred to such works as that of Weinmann and Sicher (1955).

There are two types of osteogenesis—endochondral and intramembranous. In both, specialized cells are concerned with bone formation and removal. The former cells, osteoblasts, can be seen to take on this function, especially in the early states of intramembranous bone formation. They are usually cubical or flattened cells, with cytoplasm staining strongly with basic dyes, and lie in a row along the face of the bone they are forming. Several of them become included in bone matrix and are then called osteocytes. The bone-removing cells are called osteoclasts.

In general it is agreed that all bone cells spring from a common ancestor, and that they can revert to a more primitive form and change one into another. Bloom _et al._ (1958) first developed this thesis and emphasized that mitoses were never seen. Tonna and Cronkite (1961) concluded that osteogenic cells were a self-sustaining, relatively quiescent population, osteoblasts being produced from preosteoblasts. Young (1962) developed this concept further in defining osteoprogenitor cells from which specialized bone cells arose. Osteoclasts formed from fusion of osteoprogenitor cells. Scott (1967) considered that there were two pathways of specialization of bone cells, into osteoblasts or osteoclasts, but this view is not generally held.

In intramembranous bone formation, lime salts are laid down directly on a matrix of collagen fibers, glycosaminoglycans, and lipids, the appositional side of the bone being lined with osteoblasts and the resorptive side with osteoclasts upon it. The calcified bone is always covered by a thin layer of uncalcified tissue, the preosseous matrix.

Endochondral ossification usually is seen at the ends of long bones. Here a cartilage matrix is first used as a scaffold for the formation of the primary spongiosa. Concurrently the shaft increases in width and thickness by processes of intramembranous ossification and resorption. Endochondral ossification is mainly concerned with bone growth. The cartilage cells of the growth plate pass through various stages till they finally mature and are eroded by capillaries (Dodds and Cameron, 1934). The growth plate can be divided into four zones. Resting cells form a narrow layer, followed by the proliferative phase, a wide zone where the cells become thicker and finally square in profile. Next is the hypertrophic layer where the cells become large and translucent in appearance. These cells contain glycogen and calcification starts in the longitudinal walls between the cell columns. It is this zone that becomes wide in rickets. The last zone, that of cartilage removal, is characterized by erosion by capillaries, which remove the transverse bars between the cells. Calcification is usually four cells ahead of capillary invasion. Eeg-Larsen (1956) reported that in young rats each cartilage cell took from 30 to 45 hours in its movement from the cell-dividing zone to its disappearance in the calcifying area. During the process of erosion, longitudinal cartilage trabeculae are overlaid with bone to form the primary spongiosa, which is remodeled to form a stronger structure, the secondary spongiosa which blends with the shaft.

The process of capillary erosion has been studied in some detail since it appears that cartilage may not be removed by giant cells (Cameron, 1961) but possibly by cells arising from the capillary endothelium

(Trueta, 1963; M. H. Irving, 1964) which may also be the parent cells of osteoblasts (Mankin, 1964). Anderson and Parker (1966) considered that phagocytic cells preceded the capillary endothelium and were the active eroding elements. Schenk et al. (1967) believe two mechanisms are involved, the perivascular cells removing transverse cartilage bars, and chondroclasts dealing with calcified longitudinal trabeculae. Sledge and Dingle (1965) noted that high oxygen tensions caused the release of lysosomal enzymes from cartilage cells, and speculated that this phenomenon might be a factor in the resorption of cartilage in the presence of capillaries.

The cartilage of articular surfaces and the mandibular condyle have a superficial resemblance to growth plates but they have little to do with growth of bone, and their development is in many ways quite dissimilar (Durkin et al., 1971).

With the cessation of growth, the epiphysis closes and the cartilage disappears. The formation of bone and exchange of bone salts, however do not stop with the cessation of growth. Bone is a most labile tissue, and in spite of its apparent fixity of structure, remodeling and replacement go on continuously.

Bone Resorption

Bone resorption is carried out by osteoclasts, which are large cells with many nuclei, usually about six, and the cytoplasm under the light microscope takes up acidic stains in a characteristic way. Under the electron microscope they can be seen to possess a ruffled border against the bone that is being resorbed, often causing the appearance of Howship's lacunae. Compared with osteoblasts, which line the bone face in a continuous row, osteoclasts are seen less frequently, but they have been shown to be motile (Hancox, 1949).

Evidence has also been produced that blood cells may be the parents of osteoclasts (Fischman and Hay, 1962; Gillman and Wright, 1966). Irving and Migliore (1965) found bone-resorbing giant cells to arise from fusion of mesenchymal cells. While the parent cells of osteoclasts are not definitely determined, there is no doubt that these cells arise from fusion of other cells. Bélanger et al. (1966) have produced evidence that osteocytes also have an osteolytic function.

Osteoclasts are under the direct control of the parathyroid hormone and of calcitonin, and are probably governed by other factors as yet unknown.

The ruffled border is a specialized structure concerned with resorption of bone and cartilage. Scott and Pease (1956) reported that mineral crystals were phagocyted through the ruffled border and digested in vacuoles. Hancox and Boothroyd (1961) described pinocytotic granules containing bone salt crystals, the folds of the ruffled border containing crystals and collagen fibrils. Initially collagen fibrils became separated from each other and bone salt crystals became detached. Later, as crystals and ground substance disappeared, the outline and cross-striation of the collagen fibrils became distinct.

This raises the question, possibly now rather academic, as to which process is first, crystal removal or collagen degradation. It would be expected on theoretical grounds that crystal removal should precede, since bone collagen is not available to reaction with such reagents as fluorodinitrobenzene until decalcification has at least started (Solomons and Irving, 1958). However, largely on electron microcopic grounds, Scott and Pease (1956) and Gonzales and Karnovsky (1961) reported that dissolution of collagen fibrils preceded phagocytosis of the crystals by osteoclasts. On the other hand, Takuma (1962) believed that the inorganic phase was first removed, since collagen fibrils, denuded of crystals, could be seen at the bone edge in his electron micrographs. Yaeger and Kraucunas (1969) reported the same in bone resorption in frogs. Dudley and Spiro (1961) found no unmineralized collagen at the resorption sites and concluded that mineral and organic phase removal must be about simultaneous. Bohatirchuk (1966) considered that a two-stage process occurred, first "calciolysis," the decalcified matrix being then invaded by phagocytes and resorbed.

It has been found by several workers that older bone is more readily resorbed than that recently laid down. This was reported by Harrison and Fraser (1960), by Woods (quoted in Nichols, 1963), and most recently by Irving and Heeley (1970b), who used a bone implantation technique. They reported that giant cells could not remove labeled hydroxyproline from the collagen of bone laid down 6 hours before, but would do so some days later, though in the latter case they did not phagocyte the label. Irving and Heeley suggested that preosseous matrix might be a protective layer, since Irving and Handelman (1963) had previously reported, using the same technique, that giant cells did not attack uncalcified rachitic osteoid. The same apparently applies in teeth. Selzer *et al.* (1963) found in pulp inflammation that dentin could be resorbed, but predentin only with difficulty.

APATITE CRYSTAL REMOVAL

The factors responsible for the removal of both phases have been considerably investigated. Walker (1961) reported that osteoclasts were lacking in isocitric dehydrogenase, and suggested that citric acid was the agent removing apatite crystals. Unfortunately for this theory, both Fullmer (1964) and Handelman *et al.* (1964) could not confirm Walker's finding, Handelman *et al.* reporting the presence of a large number of the enzymes of the Kreb's cycle in these cells. However, evidence from other sources does strongly suggest that citric acid may be implicated. Kenny *et al.* (1959), using bone organ culture, found citric acid to be produced during resorption, 8 to 19 times as much being produced as was present in the original calvaria. Mecca *et al.* (1963) reported, again using organ culture systems, that citrate production more closely paralleled mineral dissolution, lactic acid production merely correlating with an increased glucose utilization. Nisbet *et al.* (1970) stated that while citrate correlated best with calcium resorption, too little was produced to account for all the resorption on a molar basis. Vaes (1968b) considered, however, that the total acid released (citric plus lactic) could account for the resorption of all the mineral. Citrate is an attractive candidate for apatite crystal removal, as its well-known chelating action would not require much of a drop in pH for the removal of calcium salts. It may be considered the favorite at the moment.

COLLAGENASE

The removal of collagen by a substance dissolving the protein was suggested by Scott and Pease (1956) and by Gonzales and Karnovsky (1961). The difficulty in isolating and identifying a bone collagenase is apparently owing to the fact that osteoclasts do not store the enzyme. Woods and Nichols (1963) incubated bone cells with pure labeled bone collagen and found radioactivity to be released, the action being abolished by heating the bone homogenate. Walker *et al.* (1964)

described a collagenolytic factor in bone which was greatly increased by giving parathyroid hormone to the animal before removal of the bone, and Shimizu *et al.* (1969), using Goldhaber's bone organ culture system, succeeded in isolating collagenase from the culture medium. They found it to have an optimum pH of 7.8 to 8.0, not to be lysosomal in origin, and to cleave the collagen macromolecule into two fragments, which Gross and Nagai (1965) had also found to be the action of tadpole tail collagenase.

ACID PHOSPHATASE

Another enzyme which is associated with osteoclasts and bone resorption is acid phosphatase; it almost is a "trademark" of osteoclasts and bone-resorbing cells when studied histochemically, Susi *et al.* (1966) finding its presence to correlate with resorption and osteoclast activity. Handelman *et al.* (1964) found the enzyme not only in osteoclasts but also as a concentrated rim at the junction of osteoclast and bone, which was also reported by Wergedal and Baylink (1969). Irving and Bond (1968) studied subcutaneous autogenous implants of decalcified molar teeth, and reported that the dentin was rapidly invaded and destroyed by small round cells which were also very active in acid phosphatase. Wergedal (1970) has reported that there are two acid phosphatases in bone: one, a nonspecific enzyme similar to that found in liver lysosomes, and the other, assayed with phenylphosphate, having properties similar to those of phosphoprotein phosphatase. It is thus of interest that Kreitzman and Fritz (1970) have suggested that phosphoprotein phosphatase, which removes phosphate from phosphoproteins, acts in conjunction with collagenase in bone resorption *in vitro*; if the two enzymes are identical, this may account for the presence of acid phosphatase in bone-resorping cells.

As mentioned earlier, Bélanger and his colleagues (1966) suggested that osteocytes had an osteolytic function, and were under the control of the parathyroid gland. They considered these cells to be concerned in the maintenance of calcium homeostasis, but osteoclasts to have a specialized function in the presence of abnormal skeletal material, and to be concerned with the maintenance of the integrity of the body. A similar concept has been enunciated by MacGregor (1964), who considered osteoclast action to be slow compared to that of osteocytes.

_____ *Chapter 9*

BONE

Chemical Composition of Bone

The principal constituents of bone are inorganic salts, proteins, glycosaminoglycans, lipids, and water. Basically the composition is as shown in the following tabulation (Wuthier, 1968).

Constituent	Percent
Water	30.3
Ash	42.1
Organic material (nondialyzable)	18.7

In dry fully calcified fat-free bone, the ash content is approximately 65%, but varies somewhat from bone to bone (Trotter and Peterson, 1955). The percentages of calcium and phosphorus are around 26.7 and 12.5, respectively (Armstrong and Singer, 1965). Pugliarello *et al.* (1970) reported that if fully calcified bone be regarded at 100%, osteoid was 11.65% calcified, and osteones at the lowest degree of calcification were

50.5% calcified. About 90% of the organic matter is collagen (Eastoe, 1956), 9.5% mucosubstances (G. M. Herring, private communication), and 0.6% lipid (Wuthier, 1968). In an electron probe analysis of the mandible, Green et al. (1970) reported the following: calcium 26–32%, phosphorus 12–15%, and Ca/P molar ratio 1.56–1.68.

The Apatite Crystals of Bone

SIZE OF THE CRYSTALS

These crystals are submicroscopic and can be visualized only with the electron microscope. There is general agreement as to their dimensions but not complete agreement about their shape. Speckman and Norris (1957) saw them as groups of bundles 50 Å thick and 600–700 Å long, rod- or needle-shaped, occupying about 40% of the volume of the tissue. Carlström and Glas (1959) used line broadening measurements on oriented specimens of fish bone, which are more reliable than X-ray data. They found the crystals to be long rods; average diameter, 40–50 Å; and average length, 600–700 Å. Myers and Engström (1965) studied the crystals in calcifying turkey tendons, using X-ray diffraction and electron microscopy and found a length of 300–400 Å, and, assuming no strain, a diameter of about 60 Å. Although most workers agree that the crystals are needles rather than plates, Robinson and Watson (1952) had earlier described them as plates. Johansen and Parks (1960) developed a technique for tilting sections under the electron microscope; when this was done, crystals which appeared as needles in one plane sometimes became platelike in another. Similar results have been reported by Bocciarelli (1970). Holmes et al. (1970) found the surface of bone crystals in two samples to be 182 and 200 m²/g.

Molnar (1960) studied the growth of crystals during the mineralization of bone in vivo, using the electron microscope. She noted that the first microcrystals were about 30 × 50 Å and that these grew so that final length of 50–1000 Å was attained, some rods being as long as 3000–4000 Å. All, however, exhibited subunits of 50 Å. She therefore concluded that the crystals were formed of chains of microcrystals in an end-to-end relationship. Since the other methods used presumably gave a statistical value for the length of the crystals it is indeed possible that individual crystals have a variety of length.

CHEMISTRY OF THE APATITE CRYSTALS

The formula of hydroxyapatite is $Ca_{10}(PO_4)_6(OH)_2$, with a Ca/P molar ratio of 1.67, this formula being that of the unit cell. This cell has been defined as follows by McLean and Urist (1961): "It is the smallest expression of the ions found in the same ratios and in the same spatial relationship in which they are present throughout the entire crystal. Imaginary lines, connecting the ions, drawn in an arbitrary but regular way, outline the unit cell. When extended through the crystal structure they result in a three-dimensional lattice—the *crystal lattice*." In a cross section of the crystal, the unit is a two-dimensional parallelogram with four equal sides 9.4 Å long, and this is the α-axis of the cell. When viewed in three dimensions, the unit cell is a six-sided right prism, the other dimension or c-axis measuring 6.9 Å. This c-axis is oriented in the long dimension of the bone salt crystal. It has been found that 47.5% of the unit cells are on the surface of the crystal and about 6% of these cells have two faces exposed.

Neuman and Neuman (1958) postulated that the crystal, being in a watery medium, had four regions: the crystal interior, the crystal surface, hydration layer beyond the surface, and a weakly held oriented boundary layer which bordered the true solution phase. In such a system ion exchange can occur readily. This process is defined as a movement of ions between two masses or compartments of a pool, without detectable change in mass or compartment size (Aubert *et al.* 1963). When ions normally present exchange, this is called isoionic exchange; and with ions normally not present, the process is heterionic exchange.

With synthetic apatite crystals, the following sequence of events is possible: (1) Ions may diffuse into the hydration layer but not concentrate there. This is a reversible state, can be attained in a few hours, and the ion concentration in the hydration layer is proportional to the ion concentration in solution. Monovalent ions are examples of this class. (2) Ions can enter the hydration layer and tend to concentrate there participating in the neutralization of the charge asymmetry of the surface area of the apatite crystals; this reaction usually involved multivalent ions and the steady state of this reaction is achieved in a few hours. (3) Ions can pass through the hydration layer and exchange with ions on the crystal surface; this is a reversible reaction and equilibrium is attained in a few hours. (4) Ions in the crystal interior may be replaced by ions from the solution; this reaction takes a long time and is apparently irreversible.

It should be stressed however that these properties apply to apatite crystals in an *in vitro* medium..Neuman *et al.* (1968) and Triffitt *et al.* (1968), using the "cycling time" method, found that in comparison with many ions such as sodium, chloride, and potassium, calcium and phosphorus had a minimal exchange rate; they queried the validity of "available" and "unavailable" skeleton, since this depended on the ion and conditions being studied. Rowland (1966) had found that less than 0.2% of bone calcium was exchangeable *in vivo* and Holmes *et al.* (1970) suggest that collagen *in vivo* can screen the surface of bone mineral from body fluids. Earlier, Dallemagne *et al.* (1955) had found that only a fraction of the calcium bound to phosphate or carbonate could act as a mobilizable store and be exchanged, and Arnold *et al.* (1956) reported that the fixation of ^{45}Ca in bone was rapid and virtually irreversible.

De Jong in 1926 established with X-ray diffraction studies that the major constituent of all mineralized tissues was an apatite, but ions other than those in the formula given above are often found in the inorganic portion of bone and teeth. Certain ions (e.g., fluorine and strontium) can exchange with ions on the apatite lattice without altering the crystal charge.

Changes in the molar Ca:P ratio of biologically occurring apatites have been frequently observed, the figure usually being lower than the theoretical value of 1.67. It has been claimed by some workers (e.g., Pellegrino and Biltz, 1968) that ratios higher than this can be found in bone, but this has never been found in any bone, of any age, by the group associated with the present writer.

Apatites with a Ca/P molar ratio less than 1.67 will yield pyrophosphate when heated to about 500°C. When heated above this point the pyrophosphate disappears and is replaced by β-tricalcium phosphate (Winand, 1961), and the lower the Ca/P ratio, the more pyrophosphate is formed (Herman *et al.*, 1961).

It is postulated that apatites with a lower Ca/P ratio contain acidic phosphate groups, HPO_4^{2-}, in the lattice, and pyrophosphate is formed on heating owing to dehydration and condensation. Thus this estimation can be used as an index of the number of acidic phosphate groups present.

Lowering of the Ca:P ratio was at one time thought to be due to adsorption of phosphate on the crystal surface. However, Winand (1961) has calculated that not enough surface is present on hydroxyapatite crystals to lower the ratio from 1.67 to 1.50. Present views are that calcium-deficient apatites exist and three theories have been stated: One, that calcium ions are missing from the crystal surface and are replaced with hydronium ions, H_3O^+, to maintain charge neutrality (Neuman and Neuman, 1953). However, this theory implies the absence of HPO_4^{2-} groups, but since pyrophosphate is formed on heating (Gee and Dietz, 1955) it cannot be correct. In addition hydronium has never been detected in bone. The other two views suggest the absence of calcium from the apatite lattice. Posner and his school (Posner and Perloff, 1957) proposed that calcium was statistically missing from the crystal, the charge neutrality being maintained by hydrogen bonds between orthophosphate groups surrounding the defects. This would explain the presence of HPO_4^{2-} groups as found by Gee and Dietz.

The third theory is that of Brown *et al.* (1962), who suggested that the calcium-deficient apatites were actually lamellar intergrowths of octacalcium phosphate $[Ca_8H_2(PO_4)_6 \cdot 5H_2O]$ and hydroxyapatite. This concept would explain Ca/P ratios lower than 1.67, and this mixture will in fact produce pyrophosphate on gentle healing. However, while octacalcium phosphate is a well-recognized compound, it has never been detected in bone or tooth apatites, but it has been found in dental calculus (Rowles, 1958) and in renal stones (MacGregor *et al.*, 1965), in the latter case as a surface structure and in small amounts. Thus whatever the explanation of Ca/P ratios lower than the theoretical, the fact remains that in bone mineral such ratios have been found.

It has further been suggested that recently formed bone has a mineral with a lower Ca/P ratio, which increases as the bone becomes more mature. MacGregor and Brown (1965) think that this is octacalcium phosphate. It must be stated, however, that there still seems to be some disagreement on this point. Vincent *et al.* (1965) used quantitative autoradiography of neutron-activated sections of bone at different stages of mineralization and concluded that the Ca/P ratio remained constant as mineralization was completed. Strandh (1960) separated osteones of varying degrees of mineralization by microdissection, the degree of mineralization being gauged by microradiography. All osteones and lamellar bone examined had a Ca/P weight ratio of 2.221 ±

0.001, which is very close to the theoretical for hydroxyapatite. Alcock and Reid (1969) reported similar findings. However, since bone apatite always yields some pyrophosphate on heating, it must be assumed that extra calcium was present, possibly as carbonate.

Ibsen and Urist (1964) injected rabbits of different ages with oxytetracycline (which is taken up by newly formed bone), ground the bone, and separated the fluorescent from the nonfluorescent particles. They found that the fluorescent bone yielded much more pyrophosphate on heating than did the nonfluorescent fraction, and also that the bones of younger animals gave more pyrophosphate than those of older animals. François (1961) had earlier found that bone from newborn rats formed more pyrophosphate on heating than that from older animals and Wuthier (in Termine et al., 1967b) reported that the Ca/P ratio of epiphyseal cartilage ash rose, as one proceeded down the plate from 1.48 in the hypertrophic-proliferating zone, to 1.56 in calcified cartilage and 1.62 in cancellous bone. In rickets, a bone was produced that yielded more pyrophosphate than normal (Muller et al., 1966) and low calcium diets lowered the Ca/P ratio of bone ash from 1.58 to 1.47. The latter work was done on piglets and the bone ash of the normal animals was only 48% (Miller et al., 1962).

On the balance of the evidence, it appears that a less "mature" apatite is laid down in young bone, and that it changes with time to hydroxyapatite with 9 or 10 calcium ions in the lattice. Bone whose calcification has been interfered with also has a less mature apatite. However, since bone of any age will yield some pyrophosphate, the ideal formula is presumably never achieved.

AMORPHOUS CALCIUM PHOSPHATE

Many electron microscopists had noted a haze around the calcification front (e.g., Robinson and Watson, 1955; Hancox and Boothroyd, 1965); Molnar (1959) described the presence of dense circles or ovals 60–200 Å in diameter. At about that time Eanes et al. (1965) studied the preparation and physicochemical behavior of metastable amorphous calcium phosphate. They found that the amorphous precipitate redissolved and then crystallized out as apatite, by means of an autocatalytic kinetic mechanism. The synthetic amorphous particles had an electron microscopic appearance very similar to that described by

Molnar. Quantative X-ray diffraction analysis revealed that both amorphous and crystalline calcium phosphate salts were present in mineralizing tissues, the amorphous material probably being a hydrated tricalcium phosphate (Eanes and Posner, 1968; Eanes, 1970). Harper and Posner (1966) found in adult bone from several species that about 40% of the mineral was noncrystalline. Termine *et al.* (1967b) studied the proportion of the two forms in fetal calf growth plate and bone, and found that the amount of amorphous calcium phosphate as a percentage of the total calcium phosphate fell from 50% in the hypertrophic-proliferating zone to 32% in calcified cartilage and was at a similar level, 33%, in compact bone.

Thus it seems probable that the earliest mineral to be deposited is the amorphous form and that this is converted to crystalline bone apatite by a process similar to that observed *in vitro*. Presumably some regulatory mechanism must exist which allows the amorphous salt to persist in mature bone tissue and which controls its conversion into apatite crystals. Such a mechanism has been postulated by Fleisch *et al.* (1968), who have shown that pyrophosphate will delay this transformation *in vitro*.

CARBONATE APATITE

Sobel *et al.* (1945) showed some time ago that the CO_3/P ratio of bone ash was influenced by the Ca/P ratio of the diet. The question has often been debated since then as to whether carbonate ions can substitute in the apatite crystal. McConnell (1955) has long held this view and instanced the apatite mineral francolite which contains carbonate and shows no calcium or magnesium carbonate as a separate phase. He thought that carbonic anhydrase was involved in bone formation (McConnell *et al.*, 1961) but this has not been confirmed by others. In 1960 McConnell reported that enamel apatite was a single mineral phase, carbonate apatite, and saw no reason to suppose that the chemistry of bone or dentin mineral should be different.

In spite of views swinging one way or the other, more recent work has tended to support McConnell's thesis. Simpson (1965) found that the hydroxy and carbonate apatites had virtually the same a_0 and c_0 dimensions. A deficiency in calcium or phosphorus in carbonate apatite suggested a coupled substitution of hydronium and carbonate ions in the crystal structure. Neuman and Mulryan (1967) made synthetic carbonate apatite crystals which had a single phase. 60% of the CO_2 was within the crystal lattice, presumably as CO_3^{2-}, and 40% presumably as HCO_3^- resided in the hydration shell. Of the latter about half was lost on drying. Young rats bones were labeled with labeled CO_2, and about half of the CO_2 of these bones was lost in drying, so their model appeared to be biologically applicable. Pellegrino and Biltz (1968) analysed the bones of different animals and found a linear relationship between the Ca/P molar ratio and the CO_3 content of the ash. They proposed this formula, $Ca_9(PO_4)_6 \cdot CaCO_3$, calcium in excess of this formula existing as a separate phase. This formula may explain the old findings of Logan and Taylor (1938), who washed bone salt with small amounts of HCl and were able to extract progressively more calcium than was contained in tricalcium phosphate, the Ca/P ratio being lowered by successive acid washings. Scharf et al. (1969), however, considered that carbonate, present in apatite to a concentration of 2%, substituted for phosphate groups. Neuman and Mulryan (1968) reported an interesting observation in this connection. Fish have a low HCO_3^- content in their blood, but their apatite has the same CO_2 content as that of mammals. Synthetic apatite crystals made under the same conditions of temperature, μ, and HCO_3^- as fish blood had only one seventh to one eighth of the CO_2 content of fish bone. Thus the composition of the fluids in bone, does not reflect in a simple way the composition of circulating plasma.

One can conclude that there is now strong evidence that carbonate apatite exists as a single phase in bone, but the position of the ion in the crystal lattice is not yet decided.

Organic Constituents of Bone

COLLAGEN

The collagen macromolecule is a fibrous protein consisting of three separate polypeptide chains, each of which is present as a left-handed spiral around its own axis. The entire macromolecule consists of these three chains which have a right-handed helix about the common axis of the macromolecule, the polypeptide chains being bound by hydrogen bonds. From the chemical viewpoint, collagen is characterized by the absence of certain amino acids, and the presence of others in large amounts. Cystine and tryptophan are absent, hydroxyproline and hydroxylysine are almost exclusively found in collagen, and glycine is found in the largest amounts, followed by proline. Methionine and tyrosine groups, on the other hand, are very infrequent.

The three polypeptide chains differ in their amino acid composition and different combinations are found in various tissue. Most collagens (e.g., of bone and skin) contain two chains of the so-called α 1 designation and one of the α 2 type (Piez et al., 1963). However more recent work (e.g., Miller et al., 1971) has shown that another chain exists, α 1 (II), and that the collagen of newborn human epiphyseal cartilage contains all of this type, while newborn skin is a mixture of $(\alpha \ 1I)_2 \ \alpha$ 2 and $(\alpha \ 1 \ III)_3$, the latter being another chain peculiar to this skin.

The formation of hydroxyproline takes place after incorporation of proline into the polypeptide chain. Gould and Woessner (1957) showed that after 7 days the collagen of the skin of scorbutic guinea pigs was grossly deficient in hydroxyproline. On administration of ascorbic acid, there was a rapid production and incorporation of this amino acid. It has now been shown that the production of hydroxyproline is caused by an enzyme, collagen proline hydroxylase (Hutton et al., 1967; Kivirikko and Prockop, 1967). This enzyme requires several cofactors, one of which is ascorbic acid, which is at last given a role in collagen synthesis. The substrate on which the enzyme acts is called protocollagen, in which hydroxyproline is present in significantly reduced amounts. Lysine is similarly hydroxylated by an enzyme.

When collagen is extracted from soft tissue, such as skin, it is found that there is a neutral salt-soluble fraction, which is that first laid down, and then passes into a citrate-soluble fraction; finally stable insoluble collagen is formed, in which there are many cross-links between the macromolecules, probably by covalent bonds. In general, bone collagen is very difficult to extract and reconstitute.

Collagen is made by a number of cells derived from mesenchyme, fibroblasts, osteoblasts, chondroblasts, and odontoblasts. Revel and Hay (1963) followed the fate of labeled proline in chondroblasts, using electron microscopy and autoradiography, and found that the labeled material was first associated with the cisternae of the endoplasmic reticulum, and shortly thereafter was found in the Golgi zone. About 2 hours later the labeled material was discharged from vacuoles into the

extracellular space, probably as tropocollagen, which then poly-
merized into striated collagen fibrils. They emphasized that collagen
fibrils did not arise from excortication and appositional growth of
fibrils originating from the ectoplasm of the cells. There is no doubt that
collagen formation by other cells follows a similar pattern. Carneiro
and Leblond (1959) earlier had put forward a similar concept, that
osteoblasts and odontoblasts elaborated a matrix precursor in their
cytoplasm which was secreted out of the cell to become collagen fibers
of bone or dentin.

The urinary excretion of hydroxyproline has been studied by a
number of workers who have considered this to be an index of collagen
turnover, the literature having been summarised by Prockop and
Kivirikko (1968). It appears that as far as bone is concerned, a considerable amount of collagen, up to 55% synthesized, is rapidly removed
from the tissue, possibly before incorporation with the calcified
material (Lapière *et al.*, 1965). Similar evidence was found from *in vitro*
studies by Golub *et al.* (1968), who considered hydroxyproline release
to be more an index of bone synthesis than degradation; Krane *et al.*
(1970) likewise considered urinary polypeptides containing hydroxyproline to be related to collagen synthesis.

Under the electron microscope, the collagen fibril is seen to have a
major striation occuring at 640 Å intervals, as well as other finer bands.
These divisions of the periodic structure correspond to the presence of
various amino acid side chains at intervals along the macromolecule.

GLYCOSAMINOGLYCANS

The glycosaminoglycans found in bone as well as in most connective
tissues consist of a repeating series of alternating glucuronic acid and
hexosamine units. Hyaluronic acid is a polymer of acetyl glucosamine
and glucuronic acid. In chondroitin sulfate the sugar is galactosa-
mine, and in addition a hydrogen sulfate group is present on each
hexosamine unit, making the compound highly acidic. Chondroitin
sulfates A and C are very similar in structure. Sialic acid has a terminal
N-acetylneuraminic acid.

Most glycosaminoglycans do not exist free, but in combination with
protein, as mucoprotein. Besides chondroitin sulfuric acid, three such
protein–carbohydrate complexes have been described in bone (Her-

ring, 1964): alkali-soluble, alkali-insoluble, and sialoprotein. G. M. Herring (private communication) has found the bone organic matrix to contain about 9.5% of mucosubstances, of which 0.7–0.8% of the matrix was chondroitin sulfate, and a small amount of hyaluronic acid. The three glycoprotein fractions made up to 8.7% of the matrix. Sialoprotein was acidic in nature due to the presence of sialic acid and glutamic and aspartic acids, and stained strongly with the periodic acid–Schiff method. Wuthier (Irving and Wuthier, 1968) found the hexosamine content of epiphyseal cartilage and bone to fall in amount as calcification proceeded. As a percentage of the organic matrix, resting cartilage had 10.4 and hypertrophic cartilage 11.4, but calcified cartilage only 5.5 and cancellous bone 1.3. As will be stated below, the glycosaminoglycans have been implicated by some workers in the calcification mechanism.

LIPIDS

While bone and growth cartilage contain only small amounts of lipid, there has recently been interest in their role in the calcification process. Leach (1958) and Zambotti et al. (1962) have reported on the lipid content of these tissues, and Enlow and Conklin (1964) and Enlow et al. (1965) described the distribution of lipids in bone. The most complete analysis has been carried out by Wuthier (1968), whose findings will be described in more detail below, but may be summarized as follows. The total growth plate contained 76.1 mg/100 g dry weight of lipid, cancellous bone 6.1 mg; and compact bone 13.2 mg; 90% of the lipids were neutral and could be extracted before demineralization of the tissue. Acidic phospholipids containing serine or inositol could be extracted only after demineralization. The extraction of acidic lipids was closely related to the degree of mineralization and it was thought possible that they formed part of a lipoprotein–mineral complex in the calcifying matrix.

Theories of Mineralization

Many theories explaining this phenomenon have been enunciated over the years since Robison (1923) first described alkaline phosphatase in bone and postulated that it had a role in mineralization.

Rather than mention all the subsequent theories in historical sequence, it has seemed more logical to consider the most recent findings, which are of considerable interest, and then see how the earlier work fits in with these data.

Since blood plasma and matrix fluid of epiphyseal cartilage are considered to be undersaturated in calcium and phosphate ions with respect to the formation of bone apatite (Howell *et al.*, 1968), either some mechanism for locally raising the concentration of these ions must exist, or else nucleating sites are present which would lower the energy barrier to precipitation, so that this could occur at the existing plasma calcium and phosphate levels; or else some other calcium salt is first formed, as has been suggested by Termine *et al.* (1967b).

Cellular Activity in Mineralization

Whereas earlier work tended to stress the physicochemical aspects of apatite deposition by a process of epitaxy on to an organic matrix, more recently interest has centered on the cellular level. It is well known that mitochondria will accumulate calcium in *in vivo* and *in vitro* systems (Engstrom and DeLuca, 1964; Carafoli and Lehninger, 1971) and Shapiro and Greenspan (1969) suggested that mitochondria of bone-forming cells could produce a local rise in the levels of mineral ions together with a matrix which was capable of being mineralized. Lehninger (1970) made a similar suggestion, postulating that micro-packets of amorphous calcium phosphate were released from the cell and diffused to specific calcifying sites. Matthews *et al.* (1968) found that ^{45}Ca concentrated over the cells of the growth plate, especially in the immediate vicinity of the calcification front. Later, label was found in increasing amounts over the matrix of the mineralizing zones. They considered that the calcium was first ionic, then bound, and finally extruded in an amorphous form, a concept similar to that of Termine *et al.* (1967b). Martin and Matthews (1969) extended these observations, finding ^{47}Ca in the endoplasmic reticulum and most mitochondria in the chondrocyte, the concentration increasing from the proliferative zone to that of provisional calcification. Matthews *et al.* (1968) had previously suggested that the cartilage cell acted as a calcium-binding and concentrating system. The membranes concerned with calcium binding had been associated by previous workers with ATP, mucopolysaccharides, and phosphatases, and might be the site for primary nucleation.

In 1970 Matthews *et al.* reported that while there was a gradient of mitochondria containing inorganic granules up to the zone of provisional calcification, at this level they disappeared, possibly due to the onset of calcification. In rickets, on the other hand, only a few granules were seen in the mitochondria near the zone of provisional calcification. Giving inorganic phosphate or vitamin D restored the normal density and distribution of the granules. They proposed that in low phosphate, vitamin D-deficient rickets, the mitochondria were unable to form granules, and an apatite-binding material and inorganic phosphate were needed for this process.

Both Kashiwa (1968) and Rolle (1969), using Kashiwa's glyoxal bis (2-hydroxyanil) (GBHA) method, have reported the presence of calcium in osteoblasts, osteocytes, and chondrocytes. Rolle found a direct correlation between the amount of calcium in cells and the degree of mineralization of the adjacent matrix. The presence of a pyridine-resistant lipid (see Irving, 1963) correlated with the distribution of GBHA-positive material.

Of equal interest has been the report of several workers of vesicles in cartilage matrix closely associated with the onset of calcification. Bonucci (1967) found osmiophil periodic acid–Schiff-positive bodies around chondrocytes at an early stage of calcification. Mineralization began on them and they became gradually filled with crystallites. Roundish clusters formed which coalesced, surrounded the collagen fibrils, and the matrix became entirely calcified. On decalcification an organic framework was seen in place of each apatite crystallite, which might possibly have nucleated calcium salts. In a later paper (1969) he stated that the crystals were surrounded by organic ghosts with a proteinlike structure and sheathed with acid mucopolysaccharides. The globules could form from degenerated chondrocytes or from processes of normal chondrocytes (Bonucci, 1970).

Anderson (1969) has reported similar findings. Vesicles were seen in the longitudinal septa of the growth plate from the hypertrophic cells downward. They had a close association with calcification and were found in juxtaposition to needlelike structures which were identified by electron diffraction as hydroxy or fluorapatite. The vesicles survived decalcification unlike Bonucci's bodies, probably contained or were lipid, and had lipid membranes. It was considered that the vesicles might promote apatite nucleation. In a later paper (Anderson *et al.*, 1970) they extended these observations. The vesicles were at their highest concentration in the hypertrophic zone and contained the earliest recognized deposits of apatite. They contained alkaline phosphatase and ATPase, but were very low in acid phosphatase, and thus were probably not lysosomes. They might promote calcification by increasing the local calcium and phosphate ion concentrations, and since they had a membrane and ATPase, crystallization might occur through a process of active transport.

Bernard and Pease (1969), in a study of intramembranous osteogenesis, described nucleating sites for apatite as extrusions from osteoblasts into osteoid. The crystals grew, forming bone nodules which coalesced to form bone seams, the nodules containing polysaccharides. Fully formed collagen fibrils were seen between coalesced nodules, and these authors did not agree with the view that nucleation began on collagen fibrils.

Anderson *et al.* (1970) commented on the presence of lipid, especially phospholipid, which has been demonstrated by Irving (1963) and Wuthier (1968) to be present in a distribution corresponding closely to that of the pattern of calcium deposition.

POSSIBLE ROLE OF LIPIDS

The concept that lipids might be involved in calcification was first put forward by Wells (1914), but until recently little further attention was directed toward this idea except in some studies of pathological calcification. Leach (1958) reported briefly on the lipid content of untreated bovine compact bone and Zambotti *et al.* (1962) described the lipids of pig epiphyseal cartilage. Enlow and Conklin (1964) and Enlow *et al.* (1965) discussed the distribution of lipids in bone and suggested there might be a relationship between matrix lipid and the calcification process. Howell *et al.* (1965) found a significant alteration in the phospholipid pattern of costochondral plates during vitamin D deprivation and Cruess and Clark (1965, 1967) have reported an increase in phospholipid synthesis during hypervitaminosis D. Dirksen (1963), Dirksen and Ikels (1964), and Shapiro *et al.* (1966) have investigated the composition of lipids in enamel and dentin.

Irving and his group have postulated over the past few years that lipids are in some way concerned with the initiation of calcification. Current work and views are summarized in Irving and Wuthier (1968). This concept arose from the observation by Irving (1958) that after preliminary extraction with pyridine, all calcifying sites in bone and teeth stained strongly with Sudan black B. Similar results in bone have been reported by Ponlot (1960) and Rolle (1965, 1969). It was subsequently found (Irving, 1963) that other lipid stains were equally effective. Such staining disappeared during rickets (Irving, 1960) and scurvy (Irving and Durkin, 1965) but immediately reappeared after treatment of the animals with vitamin D or ascorbic acid. In addition, areas of ectopic calcification caused by calciphylaxis (Irving, 1965) or large doses of vitamin D (Irving et al., 1966) also stained strongly with Sudan black. Crenshaw and Heeley (1967) found sudanophilia in the mollusc shell during calcification. However, sudanophilia did not accompany in vitro calcification. It was not found in aortas calcified in vitro (courtesy of Dr. Schiffman), or in in vitro calcification of bone and tendon (M. R. Urist, personal communication). Thus some kind of "vital" process was involved.

It is of interest that only the area where calcification is being initiated is stained, and it appears that once calcification has begun, the lipids are removed. This is borne out by the chemical findings of Wuthier (1968) that the lipid content of cancellous bone is less than one twelfth of that of calcified cartilage. Burstone (1960) described an esterase at the junction of dentin and predentin and commented that this coincided with the site of Sudan black staining. It is possible that this is the enzyme responsible for the removal of the lipids. The pretreatment with a fat solvent is needed to "unmask" the responsible lipids. Such procedures have been described by other writers, especially Chayen et al. (1961).

Wuthier (1968) dissected the calcifying cartilage of fetal calves near term into layers and estimated the lipid content of each fraction. He found that the total lipid, expressed as a percentage of the organic matrix, increased from 1.0 in resting cartilage to 8.5 in calcifying cartilage and fell to 0.6 in cancellous bone. If the tissues were extracted before demineralization, there was little relationship between the chemical distribution of various lipids and the presence of lime salts. The acidic phospholipids, especially phosphatidyl serine and phosphatidyl inositol, were extracted in very small amounts before demineralization. After demineralization, the percentage of these two increased progressively in proportion to the degree of prior calcification, being highest in calcified cartilage. Sakai *et al.* (1969) studied the total lipid of rat long bones. They found that the total lipid of bone dropped precipitously from 10 days of age onward. The phospholipids also fell in amount but were always highest in the metaphysis during the active growth period. They speculated that this phenomenon was associated with the extremely active bone growth seen in the metaphysis.

It is significant that the sudanophil areas in the calcification front of both cartilage and bone are seen under high-power magnification to be composed of very small granules, which may be the vesicles described by Anderson and his colleagues (J. T. Irving, unpublished data).

While it seems unlikely that any one lipid was responsible for Sudan black staining, from the above evidence it would appear that the material primarily responsible was composed of acidic phospholipids. There are a number of ways these lipids could be involved in calcification. It is well known that these lipids have an affinity for cations and several writers have shown that phosphatidyl serine can bind calcium (e.g., Nash and Tobias, 1964). They may also play a role in the transport of ions across biological membranes. Thompson and De Luca (1964) and others have shown that vitamin D *in vivo* stimulates the incorporation of ^{32}P into phospholipids in various organs, and Hosoya *et al.* (1964) have found that vitamin D has both an *in vivo* and *in vitro* effect on the incorporation of serine into phosphatidyl serine of liver mitochondria. Other workers have reported similar findings.

As far as specific binding of ions is concerned, Bader (1964) found that phosphate binding by mixed phospholipids was dependent upon a prior binding with calcium ions. Hendrickson and Fullington (1965) have evidence that phosphatidyl serine acts as a tridentate ligand with alkaline earth metals such as calcium. In this way, three of the six metal coordinate bonds would be available to accept additional donor groups such as phosphate. Cotmore *et al.* (1971), using an *in vitro* biphasic system of chloroform–methanol and water, studied the calcium-binding properties of phospholipids. They found that calcium and phosphate ions formed a complex with phosphatidylserine in the form of submicroscopic spherules which contained stochiometric amounts of calcium, phosphorus, and lipid in the proportions of 12.12:6.74:1.0.

The findings cited above suggest that the lipids found by histochemical means at the calcification front may be constituents of the vesicles reported to be in this area and that they may confer on these vesicles their ability to nucleate calcium salts.

Robison's Theory

One of the earliest theories of bone calcification was suggested by Robison *et al.* (1930); they considered that a "local factor" in conjuction with alkaline phosphatase was the responsible agent. The local factor was postulated since many tissues contain alkaline phosphatase but do not calcify. The enzyme was the agent causing a local increase in phosphate ions, thus leading to the precipitation of calcium salt. This theory has been abandoned for a variety of reasons, the chief being a lack of substrates for phosphatase.

This enzyme, as far as bone is concerned, is probably more associated with matrix formation. A great deal of the earlier work tended to this view (Lorch, 1947; Siffert, 1951). Morse and Greep (1951) found in the normal epiphyseal cartilage that the content of phosphatase increased as the cells became more mature, the hypertrophic cell layer containing most, but the layer of primary calcification virtually none. In rickets the same was found in the cartilage cells, and osteoid also contained the enzyme. Danielli *et al.* (1945) studied wound healing in normal and scorbutic guinea pigs. In normal animals there were two phases of phosphatase activity in the healing tissue, one owing to leukocyte invasion, the second probably to the differentiation of collagenous fibrous tissue. But if the animal had scurvy there was no second peak and collagen formation was absent or greatly reduced. Gould and Schwachman (1942) found in scorbutic guinea pigs that the phosphatase content of serum and bone rose and fell in parallel, that of the other tissues not being significantly altered. It will be recalled that osteoblasts become inactive during scurvy forming the *gerüstmark*. During healing from scurvy the bone and blood phosphatases rose together, and Gould and Schwachman considered the blood phosphatase to be derived from osteoblasts.

Recent papers confirm these views. Wergedal and Baylink (1969) found alkaline phosphatase to be associated with osteoblasts and other mesenchymal cells at forming bone surfaces, being also present in the preosseous matrix but not at the zone of mineralization. Westmoreland and Hoekstra (1969) considered alkaline phosphatase was necessary for bone development. Strates *et al.* (1971), working with bone explants which normally calcified, found this process could be inhibited by diphosphonates. This did not prevent the appearance of alkaline phosphatase, which always accompanied the calcification process, so they concluded that there was no direct relationship between this enzyme and calcification. However, recently a new role has been suggested for the enzyme.

PYROPHOSPHATE AND CALCIFICATION

Fleisch and Neuman (1961) studied the nucleation of calcium phosphate crystals by collagen and found this process to be inhibited by a plasma ultrafiltrate, alkaline phosphatase abolishing this inhibition. Urine and plasma were found to contain crystallization inhibitors (Fleisch and Bisaz, 1962a,b), one of which was isolated and found to be inorganic pyrophosphate. The inhibiting level was too low for the effect to be due to the formation of a calcium complex and they considered crystal growth to be "poisoned." Pyrophosphate could not be used as such *in vivo*, since it was readily hydrolyzed, but Graham's salt (a long-chain polyphosphate) could be employed instead as it was resistant to enzyme attack. More recently diphosphonate, in which the oxygen linking the phosphorus atoms is replaced by a carbon atom, has been used. This compound has the advantage that it can be administered orally. Both Graham's salt and diphosphonate inhibited calcification in an organ culture system of bone and also ectopic calcification (Fleisch *et al.*, 1966; Irving *et al.*, 1966; Francis *et al.*, 1969).

The concept underlying these observations was that pyrophosphate acted as a crystal growth inhibitor by being adsorbed on the crystal face and thus preventing further growth (Fleisch, 1964). Pyrophosphatase was present in bone and thus calcification could occur. There is some argument as to whether alkaline phosphatase and pyrophosphatase are identical. Alcock and Shils (1969) found that pyrophosphatase activity increased in costal cartilage where calcification was at its height, but that there was no direct relationship between alkaline phosphatase and the onset of calcification, the two enzymes not being identical, a view also held by Berg (1964). However, Moss *et al.* (1967)

and Wöltgens *et al.* (1970) considered both activities to be due to the same enzyme. The Fleisch theory gives alkaline phosphatase a possible role in calcification. It would be satisfying if it could also explain the absence of calcification in other tissues, but, as Posner (1969) has pointed out, "Pyrophosphatase occurs ubiquitously in all tissues."

CHONDROITIN SULFATE

For many years Sobel and his associates considered chondroitin sulfate to be the chief factor involved, probably in conjunction with mucoproteins. Sobel and Burger (1954) made a collagen–chondroitin sulfate complex which took up calcium like rachitic cartilage and had a final ash content of 30% dry weight, the ash having an apatite diffraction pattern. It is of interest that metachromasia does increase in cartilage about to calcify and in areas about to become bone. Matukas and Krikos (1968) in an electron microscopic study, described protein–polysaccharide granules in epiphyseal cartilage which condensed into an amorphous electron-dense material with the onset of calcification. However, Glimcher and Krane (1962) have pointed out the danger of confusing ion binding with nucleation and thought that acid glycosaminoglycans were inhibitory to calcification. DiSalvo and Schubert (1967) extracted a protein–polysaccharide fraction from cartilage which reacted with calcium phosphate to produce a stable colloidal-calcium phosphate complex. Campo *et al.* (1969) found that protein polysaccharide extracted from articular, epiphyseal, or costal cartilage would inhibit the precipitation of calcium phosphate from solution. When the protein polysaccharide had been degraded by enzyme extracts from cartilage, this inhibitory action was lost. Both Weatherill and Weidmann (1963) and Hirschman and Dziewiatkowski (1966) showed that sulfated glycosaminoglycans or protein polysaccharides disappeared from cartilage when calcification began. Thus if these compounds had been acting as calcification inhibitors, their removal at the calcification front would be a rational event.

On the other hand, Hirschman and Silverstein (1968) carried out experiments in which glycosaminoglycan–protein complexes were removed enzymatically from rachitic epiphyseal cartilage. After this treatment, the cartilage would not calcify *in vitro*, and they considered that the removal or alteration of these complexes was not sufficient per se to make the tissue calcifiable. Using a different technique, Howell and Carlson (1968) had arrived at similar conclusions. Irving and Heeley (1970a) treated autogenous bone implants with various enzymes before implantation. Some of these enzymes abolished Alcian blue staining in the implants and these implants were invaded by capillaries and small round cells, but controls which still stained with Alcian blue were unchanged. They proposed that the role of acid glycosaminoglycans was to prevent capillary invasion in endochondral calcification. Capillary invasion is always seen in stained sections to occur at the level where these compounds disappear. On the balance of the evidence, the present writer feels that protein polysaccharides or acid glycosaminoglycans may play a regulatory role in the calcification process, but probably in association with other bone compounds.

ROLE OF COLLAGEN

Other theories of calcification involve the phenomenon of epitaxy, according to which "a parasitic phase is deposited on a host material, this in turn leading to crystal growth" (Bronner, 1964). On the basis of this theory it has been proposed that collagen is concerned in the initiation of calcification, which was first suggested by Neuman and Neuman in 1958. The present writer feels that confusion has existed between nucleation and the condition in the final calcified bone. In the latter there must be a close connection between the major organic and inorganic compounds. In fact, Marino and Becker (1967), using electron paramagnetic resonance observations, have stated that there is a direct physical binding between collagen fibers and apatite crystallites and the same conclusions, using electron spin resonance, had been reached by Termine et al. (1967a).

Wuthier et al. (1964, 1968), in an extension of the earlier work of Solomons and Irving (1958), studied the reactivity of the ε-amino groups of lysine and hydroxylysine of bone collagen using fluorodinitrobenzene. They decalcified bone, and found that four categories of amino groups became reactive. Two of these categories were associated with apatite, one being electrovalently bonded to the phosphate ions, the other category being even more strongly bonded to the mineral, and reacting with fluorodinitrobenzene only when demineralization was almost complete. The latter groups may have been bonded to pyrophosphate. Cartier and Lanzetta (1961) had also noted that during the last stages of demineralization about one third of the ε-amino groups became available to react with fluorodinitrobenzene, pyrophosphate being liberated at the same time in proportion suggesting that one molecule of pyrophosphate was bonded to two ε-amino groups.

Hodge and Petruska (1963) have described what they call their model II of collagen, which seemed to fit best with their electron microscopic images. This model predicted the presence of "holes" in the nonoverlap regions of the fibril. In embryonic bone, the initial appearance of hydroxyapatite crystals appeared to coincide with the ends of these holes in the structure.

While it is quite obvious that there must be a close relationship between the organic and mineral phases in calcified bone, the evidence that collagen is the nucleating agent does not seem to be supported by the facts. In 1956 Fitton-Jackson and Randall published electron micrographs showing the presence of submicroscopic solid aggregates on the cross-striations of collagen fibers in fowl embryo cartilage and Glimcher et al. (1957), using reconstituted collagen, found the earliest stage of calcification in vitro to be on the cross-banding. Later workers, using more modern methods, have not been able to substantiate these findings. Fernández-Morán and Engström (1957), while finding crystals aligned on the collagen periodicity of 600 Å, also found random orientation of the crystallites. Cameron (1963) and Decker (1966) studied the earliest stages of crystal formation with the electron microscope, but could not find any correlation between the first appearance of apatite crystals and collagen structure. Decker stated that "bone crystals surrounding such [collagen] fibrils are not oriented with their long axes parallel to the fibril, nor do they seem associated with either the major period or subbands of collagen." Thomas and Tomita (1967) used human tissues in in vitro calcification studies and found no relationship of collagen fibrils with apatite formation. Bernard and Pease (1969) reported that the first crystals occurred between, and not directly in association with, collagen fibrils, and stated they were unable to confirm the findings of Fitton-Jackson or Glimcher.

Glimcher and his colleagues have done much subsequent work showing that reconstituted collagen will cause crystallization of apatite, only collagen with a 640 Å axial repeat being effective

(Glimcher and Krane, 1962). François *et al.* (1967) reported phosphorus to be present in the α-chains of collagen, and postulated that this might act as the site for the heterogeneous nucleation of apatite crystals. Dentin collagen contains a set of phosphate cross-linkages distributed in specific regions of high charge density along the body of monomer units, these linkages not being found in corium collagen (Schlueter and Veis, 1964).

However, many other organic matrices will act as nucleators for apatite crystallization. In the aorta, elastin will act in this way *in vitro* (Martin *et al.*, 1963) and *in vivo* (Irving *et al.*, 1966). King and Boyce (1950) concluded from their work on renal calculus formation that calcification did not depend on any one molecular species, but that several such matrices could function in this respect. Paegle (1966) reported that the calcification in calcinosis cutis was not associated with or deposited in any morphological structure such as collagen or elastin.

Urist (1964) and his colleagues have enunciated a triphase theory that involves the reaction of calcium with "elastoid" proteins, this compound then forming a complex with phosphate. Unlike Glimcher and Krane (1962), who considered that an initial phosphate transfer occurred, Urist's concept suggests that calcium is the first ion to be involved, but it is doubtful if the data presented support the theory.

The fact that so many propositions have been put forward to explain bone mineralization shows that the solution of this problem is not yet in sight. But on the balance of the evidence, the present writer feels that investigations of the cellular reactions, described above, are the most promising approach.

Chapter 10

DIETARY FACTORS ON BONE AND CALCIUM AND PHOSPHORUS METABOLISM

Protein Uptake and Bone Formation

El-Maraghi *et al.* (1965) have emphasized that the level of protein intake is probably more important for bone formation than the level of dietary calcium. Many workers, working with rats, have shown that protein deficiency caused a gradual disappearance of the primary spongiosa and narrowing of the epiphyseal cartilage which was finally sealed off by bone (e.g., Frandsen *et al.*, 1954). The same was seen in lysine deficiency (Bavetta and Bernick, 1955; Likins *et al.*, 1957). Braham *et al.* (1961) found that lysine deficiency in chicks caused a reduction in bone protein, and Stewart and Platt (1961) described bone changes in pigs similar to those in other animals during protein deficiency.

It seems, however, that the effects of protein or amino acid deficiency are a nonspecific action on growth processes in general. Likins *et al.* (1957) reached this conclusion, and the fact that Bavetta and Bernick (1956) observed the same effects during trytophan deficiency supports this view, since this amino acid is not a constituent of collagen. Hypophysectomy, pure inanition, and deprivation of several of the B-group vitamins all caused similar bone changes (Nelson *et al.*, 1947; 1950; Silberberg and Levy, 1948). However, the bone changes during protein deficiency are not due to a reduced action of the hypophysis. Protein deficiency has no effect upon the continuously erupting incisor tooth of the rat, whereas hypophysectomy causes very profound changes in this tooth (Irving, 1956b).

Vitamin A

In deficiency of this vitamin, a curious overgrowth of bone takes place. This was first described by Moore *et al.* (1935) in calves and it was shown to be prevented by β-carotene (Moore, 1939). Wolbach (1946) considered that the normal process of bone remodeling was accentuated, but this seems improbable since new bone development can take place at sites where resorption occurs normally. Mellanby (1947) also analyzed the changes and showed that the position of osteoblasts and osteoclasts could become reversed on certain bones, and that this accounted for the development of new bone in abnormal situations. Irving (1949) considered that the action of osteoblasts became uncontrolled in the absence of vitamin A so that they formed excessive bone of a primitive type. In areas where normally resorption occurred, bone was laid down in avitaminosis A, and adjacent cells actively divided and became osteoblasts (Irving, 1956a). Frandsen and Becks (1962), on the other hand, considered that all cellular activity was depressed, leading to a failure of bone remodeling, and that the osteoclasts were especially affected (Frandsen, 1963). Gallena *et al.* (1970), working with avitaminotic calves, confirmed Irving's concept that osteoblastic activity was increased. It seems to the present writer that these different findings are probably due to different interpretations of histological appearances which are not so dissimilar.

Firschein (1970) found in avitaminotic rats that the serum calcium was unchanged, and that mineral accretion and collagen synthesis were reduced in the same proportion. In hypervitaminosis A, bone formation ceases and fractures occur (Moore and Wang, 1945), possibly owing to suppression of osteoblast activity, resorption continuing in a normal way (Irving, 1949). Barnicot (1950) found that when bone implanted into the brain was in contact with a crystal of vitamin A, resorption occurred with many osteoclasts (this action being specific to vitamin A) and proposed that the action of vitamin in excess was to cause an active resorption. Fell and Mellanby (1952), using mouse fetal bones in tissue culture, found that vitamin A in excess caused resorption of the bone but no great number of osteoclasts were present. In long bones that fracture, no particular cellular reaction is seen and it is possible that the fault lies in the organic matrix.

In 1960, Thomas *et al.* compared the histological appearances of rabbit bone after administration of papain or vitamin A in large doses. Papain, a plant proteolytic enzyme, can be injected into animals without general toxic effects. It breaks down the protein in cartilage to which acid glycosaminoglycans are attached, as a result of which the glycosaminoglycans are rapidly removed. Metachromasia is lost, the architecture of the cartilage is quite changed, and finally it disappears and is replaced by bone. Thomas *et al.*, considering that the histological changes in hypervitaminosis A were similar, postulated that the vitamin released an enzyme, similar in properties to papain, and caused the histological effects. Lucy *et al.* (1961) described an enzyme which they extracted from cartilage rudiments and which produced effects on cartilage like those of hypervitaminosis A. Irving and Rönning (1962), although not questioning the possibility of vitamin A releasing an enzyme in bone, pointed out that there was little resemblance between the histological appearances after papain injections and overdosage with vitamin A. McElligott (1962) reported that while hypervitaminosis A prevented the uptake of ^{35}S by articular and epiphyseal cartilages, papain did not, and concluded that vitamin A inhibited the synthesizing activity of the bone cell, but papain removed glycosaminoglycans from the cartilage.

Gorlin and Chaundry (1959) attributed the bone changes in hypervitaminosis A to protein deficiency caused by loss of appetite. There is a great deal of histological resemblance between the changes in the two conditions, the only doubt about this interpretation being raised by the spontaneous fractures of long bones, which occur after about 2 weeks of vitamin A overdosage, and which do not happen in protein deficiency.

Ascorbic Acid

In scurvy a very characteristic picture emerges owing to interference with the activity of the osteoblast, which modulates back to a fibroblastlike cell. A great deal of work has been done on this condition.

Delf and Tozer (1918) published an early account of experimental scurvy, and Wolbach and Howe (1926) described the changes in great detail, as has also been done by many writers since.

The chief change is an interference with ossification which leads to weakness of the bones, fractures, and infractions in areas where growth is taking place. The subsequent trauma imposed on the original pathological process gives a complicated picture that is difficult to interpret. In addition, the changes vary in different bones and in different parts of the same bone, largely as a result of the rate of bone growth and the degree to which these bones are used. For these reasons the manifestations of scurvy are more severe in growing animals than in adults.

The first change is a cessation of bone apposition. The periosteum gradually thickens, the cells composing it looking like fibroblasts. Resorption with accompanying osteoclasts continues unchanged. As a result, the shaft, especially that part at the metaphysis were remodeling normally takes place, becomes very thin and may disappear. Fracture often occurs with considerable hemorrhage and damage to the cartilage trabeculae and cell columns, producing an area of debris, hemorrhage, and fibrin deposition—the *trümmerfeld*. When this happens, the cartilage cell sequences are not so much disrupted as is capillary penetration, which is now very irregular. As the disease progresses, a mass of fibroblastlike cells develops in the metaphysis on the diaphyseal side of the *trümmerfeld*, occupying the area usually filled with the spongiosa. This zone is known as the *gerüstmark*. This mass of cells is probably made up of inactive osteoblasts that have accumulated where they would normally be calcifying the spongiosa (Wolbach and Howe, 1926). This concept is supported by the findings of rapid new calcification in the *gerüstmark* after ascorbic acid administration (Menkin *et al.*, 1934). Stunted trabeculae are produced, but this may be due to local trauma as the bone becomes weakened. Follis (1943) found that if the limb was immobilized a cartilage lattice formed but was not calcified.

The fundamental cause of these changes is still a matter of dispute, but it would probably be generally agreed that they are due to the inability of the osteoblast to secrete a calcifiable matrix. Possibly ascorbic acid has an even more fundamental action than this. In scurvy, the osteoclasts and chondroclasts, which are a prominent feature in the formation of the mandibular condyle, disappear and the condylar cartilage becomes very wide (Irving and Durkin, 1965). On administration of ascorbic acid, these cells reappear in large numbers and repair of the cartilage is complete by 72 hours. These authors thought that the differentiation of osteoprogenitor cells might be under the control of ascorbic acid.

The collagen content of bones and teeth is reduced during scurvy (Robertson, 1950), but the blood calcium and phosphate levels are unchanged (Todhunter and Brewer, 1940).

Very few biochemical effects of ascorbic acid deficiency, other than those on collagen formation mentioned above, have been reported. Banerjee and Ghosh (1961) found the hexosamine content of bones to increase in scurvy. Fullmer and Martin (1964) estimated the activity of a number of dehydrogenases in osteoblasts and odontoblasts. The only enzyme to be reduced in scurvy was $D(-)-\beta-$hydroxybutyric dehydrogenase. Thornton (1968a) produced evidence that ascorbic acid could mobilize calcium from the bones of chicks, and that the lability of bone salt of scorbutic guinea pigs was reduced *in vitro* (1968b).

Calcium, Phosphorus, and Vitamin D

If the diet is lacking in any of these, a defect in bone calcification occurs, a condition known as rickets. There is considerable species difference in the causes of this defect and it is unfortunate that rats have been so much used, since although the histological appearance is similar to that in humans and other animals, the method of producing rickets is peculiar to rodents. Rats have a very low requirement of vitamin D (Irving, 1944) and on a diet normal in calcium and phosphorus content but lacking in vitamin D, will get a marked hypocalcemia but no rickets (Harrison *et al.*, 1958). To cause rickets it is necessary to put them on a vitamin D-free diet with a low phosphorus content, with a Ca:P ratio of 4 or more. A rachitogenic diet, adequate in all other respects, had been devised recently by DeAngelis (1969). On the other hand cats (Gershoff *et al.*, 1957) and puppies (Gran, 1960) will get rickets on diets adequate in calcium and phosphorus but lacking in vitamin D. Puppies given a diet devoid of vitamin D but adequate in calcium and phosphorus grew normally but had increased amounts of unmineralized osteoid in their bone (Freeman and McLean, 1941). On a low phosphorus diet, they developed florid rickets regardless of whether or not vitamin D was given in amounts sufficient to protect puppies on an adequate mineral intake. Humans will also get rickets on diets adequate in calcium and phosphorus but lacking in vitamin D; like rats, they have a normal blood calcium, but a very low blood phosphate level (Steendijk, 1961).

Low calcium intakes produce in rats a condition histologically similar to rickets, with a low plasma calcium level, and the bone ash is considerably reduced (Boelter and Greenberg, 1941). The administration of vitamin D will prevent the pathological appearances, even if the composition of the diet is unchanged (J. T. Irving, unpublished results). Miller *et al.* (1962) found in baby pigs that a very low calcium diet reduced the bone ash from a normal figure of 48 to 29%, and the Ca/P ratio of the bone ash fell from 1.65 to 1.45.

Bauer *et al.* (1929) originally showed that the spongiosa formed a readily available store from which calcium could be withdrawn. This ability is age dependent. Old rats could withstand the adverse effects of low calcium diets, whereas young ones could not, developed skeletal lesions, and died (Moore *et al.*, 1963). Singer and Armstrong (1959) found that the fixed bone fraction was unaffected by high or low calcium diets, or low calcium diets plus vitamin D.

Histological Changes in Rickets

The prime change in endochondral ossification in rickets is an inability to calcify and erode the hypertrophic cartilage cells. There is some disagreement over which of these processes stops first. Dodds and Cameron (1934) consider failure of calcification to be the prime fault and Park also holds this view (1939). Shohl and Wolbach (1936) consider that the cartilage cells do not degenerate and thus capillary invasion, which they regard as comparable to granulation tissue formation following tissue defect, does not occur. In the early stages calcification and cartilage removal are at the same level instead of being 3 to 4 cells apart. Later, calcification of the hypertrophic cells ceases completely and with it cartilage removal. The hypertrophic cartilage cell layer becomes greatly thickened and forms a new part of the bone structure called the metaphysis, which is visible radiologically as a widened translucent zone. Osteoid is often deposited on this cartilage. Later in the condition a lawless invasion and removal of cartilage in all directions, called "resumed cartilage removal" by Dodds and Cameron, occurs, the eroded spaces being filled with twisted masses of osteoid. The rachitic metaphysis has been used by those studying the enzymatic changes in calcification, as it will recalcify *in vitro* if placed in appropriate media.

The changes in intramembranous bone during the onset of rickets have been described by Bailie and Irving (1955). The first change is a slowing of resorption, the bone gradually becoming wider. Ten days after rats had been placed on the rachitogenic diet, an osteoid margin appears on the appositional side of the bone, this margin gradually becoming wider. Between the tenth and twenty-eighth day the osteoblast, while retaining the ability to make matrix, gradually loses the power to calcify it. Resorption of the uncalcified matrix does not occur and the osteoclasts gradually disappear.

As a result of the large amount of osteoid which may be formed, the proportion of calcified mass to total mass of the bone is changed. This is usually estimated as the bone ash, which may fall from the normal value of about 65% of dry fat-free bone to less than half this figure.

Osteomalacia is a form of adult rickets. Since endochondral ossification has ceased, no epiphyseal changes are seen, but the process of calcification of replaced bone is interfered with and osteoid is laid down instead. This condition is rarely seen in Europe, but cases have been described in the Orient, especially in women after multiple pregnancies and lactations, when the skeleton has collapsed and crippled the patient.

Rickets in rats can be healed by giving vitamin D, starvation when a high Ca:P ratio diet is used (owing to mobilization of P from the soft tissues or cessation of growth), or by adjusting the Ca:P ratio of the diet. With vitamin D the classical "line" response is seen in the early stages, due to the deposition of lime salts in a line across the metaphysis, where they can be visualized with silver nitrate. Six stages of healing have been described by Coward (1938) and they form the basis of the biological estimation of the vitamin. If the animal is given extra calcium or phosphorus in the diet, healing is usually so precipitous that no line is seen, the whole metaphysis filling with calcification. The site of the line and, in fact, the development of it depends on the presence of a high degree of rickets and a great deal of "resumed cartilage removal", since calcification occurs at the edge of the epiphyseal cartilage. Exactly the same kind of calcification is seen *in vitro* if the end of the rachitic bone is incubated in a calcifying medium.

Vitamin D

ACTION ON BONE

Although as mentioned elsewhere, there is no doubt that vitamin D acts on calcium absorption in the intestine, and will also cause a rapid healing of rickets, it is still uncertain if vitamin D has a direct action on bone. Earlier work with radiocalcium and radiophosphorus showed that rachitic bone took up a great deal of both of these isotopes after D dosage (Morgareidge and Manley, 1939; Claasen and Wöstman, 1953; Greenberg, 1945; Underwood *et al.*, 1951) compared to bone of undosed animals. However, these results may be due merely to increased turnover following on increased intestinal absorption. Gaster *et al.* (1967), working with rats fed a low calcium diet, found that while vitamin D caused an increase in the uptake of ^{45}Ca, it did not alter the calcium, phosphorus, or ash content of the bone, and thus while increasing calcium turnover, did not have a calcifying effect.

Bélanger and Migicovsky (1960) thought that vitamin D stimulated the replacement and maturation of bone-forming cells and DeLuca *et al.* (1968) found, after giving labeled vitamin D_4 (an isomer), that it was present in highest amounts in bone cells (and intestinal mucosa). Anyone familiar with the histology of the healing of rickets will agree that a greater cellular change occurs in the rachitic metaphysis, capillary activity is greatly enhanced, osteoid is removed, and mature chondrocytes are formed. Krishna Rao (1961) showed that, after vitamin D dosage, amino acid changes in the epiphyseal cartilage indicated that protein was synthesized owing to vitamin D action. Furthermore, a change takes place in the enzymatic activity of the cells. Tulpole and Patwardhan (1954) reported that the epiphyseal cartilage of rachitic rats could not oxidize pyruvic acid, but that if the animals were dosed with vitamin D, this activity was restored. The ability of homogenates of liver or kidney of rachitic animals to oxidize pyruvic acid was unimpaired. Schajowicz and Cabrini (1958), working with normal rats, had found glycogen in all the cells of the epiphyseal cartilage, including the hypertrophic cells if growth was slow, but this disappeared from the hypertrophic cells if growth was fast. Dixit (1967), in a comparable way, found that the glycogen of rachitic epiphyseal cartilage fell to about half its original content if the animals were given vitamin D. Kunin and Krane (1965a) reported that aerobic glycolysis was greater in rachitic epiphyseal cartilage *in vitro* than that of normal cartilage. This was reversed by adding phosphate to the diet before the animals were sacrificed, but vitamin D did not have this effect. They attributed the lack of control of glycolysis to phosphate depletion. In a later paper (Meyer and Kunin, 1969) they reported that both vitamin D or increased dietary phosphate reduced the increase in glycolysis and glycolytic enzymes found in rachitic cartilage. Both factors likewise reduced the glycogen and protein contents of the cartilage, which were also increased during rickets. Thus it would appear that the effects of vitamin D on these changes was secondary to its effect in increasing the blood, and thus the tissue fluid, phosphate. Dixit (1969) found the levels of 6-phosphogluconic dehydrogenase and lactic dehydrogenase to be increased in rachitic rat cartilage and to be reduced both by vitamin D treatment or starvation, the latter process healing rickets by mobilizing tissue phosphate. Thus it would appear again that the action of vitamin D, at least under these conditions, could be secondary and due to changes in blood composition.

But evidence has been produced indicating that vitamin D may have a direct effect upon bone. Mankin and Lippiello (1969) found that the synthesis of RNA, protein, and polysaccharide was virtually stopped in the maturation zone in rickets (this is a narrow zone sometimes described as being between the proliferative and hypertrophic areas). On giving vitamin D, these syntheses rapidly increased in an area where calcification was not being initiated. Rasmussen (1969) placed rats on a diet adequate in all respects except vitamin D, and containing sufficient calcium and phosphate. The serum calcium fell and inorganic phosphate rose, but the product of these two ions was adequate for calcification. Nonetheless, there was a delay in the mineralization of the hypertrophic cartilage, suggesting that vitamin D was essential for this to occur. Canas et al. (1969) found that the labeling of rachitic bone with [³H] proline occurred as quickly as 12 hours after small doses of vitamin D_3 and before a rise occurred in the serum calcium. There was no change in the specific activity of skin collagen nor in the proline radioactivity of the blood. They considered the vitamin D action to be specific to bone. Thornton (1970), working with chicks, likewise felt that rachitic healing preceded the effects of vitamin D on calcium absorption in the intestine. One defect in the interpretation of some of these experiments is that the methods used for calcium and phosphate estimations may be too crude to detect minimal changes in blood composition sufficient to initiate the healing process. The ideal experiment would be to inject vitamin D into eviscerated rachitic rats, but the operative procedure would undoubtedly cause some degree of bone healing. It is, however, of interest that Kodicek and Thompson (1965) found labeled vitamin D to be taken up by the proliferative cell layer of the growth plate of rachitic rats, and not by hypertrophic chondrocytes or osteoblasts, suggesting that under these circumstances vitamin D was not so much concerned with calcification as matrix formation.

Thus, it is still impossible to decide if vitamin D has a direct calcifying action in bone, but the balance of the evidence is against this view, and the most that can be postulated is that bone shows, with the rest of the body, an increased turnover of calcium and phosphorus when vitamin D is given. As is well known, Shipley *et al.* (1926) demonstrated that rachitic epiphyseal cartilage would calcify *in vitro* in solutions of appropriate calcium and phosphate content and this has been repeatedly confirmed by others. Fraser *et al.* (1957) found that the cartilage from children with rickets would calcify *in vitro* if placed in serum from normal children, and Steendijk (1961) caused healing of rickets in a case of cystinosis by phosphate infusions. Lamm and Neuman (1958) exhaustively demineralized the epiphyseal ends of bones of rats on high-calcium, low-phosphorus diets, with and without vitamin D, and then incubated them in calcifying media. All calcified equally well and they concluded that the failure of the mineralization process in vitamin D deficiency was due to something other than an alteration in collagen structure and function. P. Rasmussen (1970) has similarly shown that vitamin D deficiency in rats did not prevent the formation of a bone matrix that could attain a normal degree of mineralization. Gran (1960) showed that injected calcium was well retained by puppies on a vitamin D-free diet.

HYPERVITAMINOSIS D

When one turns to the effects of hypervitaminosis D on bone, there is no doubt that a direct and destructive effect is observed, and this has been used clinically to cause mobilization of calcium. Large amounts of osteoid are laid down (Hass *et al.*, 1958), no bone formation occurs, and much resorption is seen (Chen and Bosmann, 1965). This is accompanied by hypercalcemia and ectopic calcification, especially in the kidney and aorta. Clark and Smith (1964) have found this effect to be largely prevented by simultaneous large doses of vitamin A. This they thought to be due to the suppression of the increased glycosaminoglycan and collagen turnover which occurs in hypervitaminosis D. Eisenstein and Passavoy (1964) found that actinomycin D inhibited the hypercalcemia of hypervitaminosis D and diminished osteoid formation, and they concluded that vitamin D could act by inducing synthesis of new enzymes via DNA directed RNA in bone, which would degrade the tissue. It is of interest in this connection that Trummel *et al.* (1969) found that although vitamin D_3 added to an organ culture of previously labeled bone had no effect upon the release of ^{45}Ca into the medium, 25-hydroxycholecalciferol in much smaller amounts would cause this. The effect was similar to that produced by parathyroid hormone with respect to time course, dose response, and inhibition by calcitonin. Thus it is possible that 25-hydroxycholecalciferol, or a similar metabolite, besides exerting its action on calcium absorption in the intestine, also initiates bone changes.

To explain the fact that growth is often decreased in rachitic animals when dosed with vitamin D, Cramer and Steenbock (1956) postulated that the vitamin could cause a transfer of phosphorus from soft tissues to bone. In puppies on a low calcium and phosphorus diet, Campbell and Douglas (1965) found that vitamin D dosage caused an osteoporosis of great severity owing to the vitamin maintaining the blood mineral levels at the expense of bone. In this case, it would be interesting to speculate that the parathyroid glands were also involved.

VITAMIN D AND CITRATE METABOLISM

Vitamin D has often been implicated in the control of bone citrate. Rachitic epiphyseal cartilage had a lowered citrate content, a depres-

sed citrate metabolism, and diminished ability to synthesize citrate
from precursors (Meyer *et al.*, 1959), DeLuca *et al.* (1961) noted that
while pantothenic acid or vitamin B_6 deficiency reduced urinary, blood,
and kidney citrate, affecting bone citrate only slightly, vitamin D deficiency lowered all three values, and bone citrate was decreased as
well. It would appear that different metabolisms were affected during
these deficiencies, since Meintzer *et al.* (1961) found the increase of
plasma calcium and citrate induced by vitamin D to be less in older
animals whose bone metabolism was presumably lessened, indicating
that the plasma citrate might come from bone. The same conclusion
can be reached from the results of Harrison *et al.* (1957), who found
that cortisol stopped the increase in both plasma and bone citrate
mediated by vitamin D, but did not prevent the rise in plasma phosphate or bone healing, and thus the two actions of the vitamin could be
separated. In a second paper (1958) they found that while cortisol
blocked the citrate action of vitamin D, it had no effect upon the eleva-
tion of serum calcium caused by the vitamin. Hartles *et al.* (1964) concluded that vitamin D had a direct effect upon citrate synthesis in bone,
but that not all the bone citrate was formed *in situ*.

Both Norman and DeLuca (1964a) and Kunin and Krane (1965b)
have studied the rate of citrate metabolism and its relation to vitamin
D. Norman and DeLuca gave labeled acetate and vitamin D to rachitic
rats and studied the effect upon the labeling of organic acids in spongiosa and trabecular bone. There was an increase in citrate compared
to undosed rats, but a decrease in activity in all the other organic acids
studied, indicating that vitamin D did not cause an increase in citrate
synthesis, but a decrease in the rate of its conversion into subsequent
intermediates of the tricarboxylic acid cycle. Kunin and Krane found
that rachitic epiphyseal cartilage utilized citrate at a greater rate than
that of normal rats or those given vitamin D or extra phosphate; they
thought the low citrate content might be due to increased utilization.
Like Norman and DeLuca, they found that vitamin D added to the diet
increased the citrate content, but it did not alter the rickets histologically, while phosphate addition had little effect upon the citrate content, but caused some histological healing.

In almost all of these experiments, prophylactic doses of vitamin D
were used, so that the effect was one that could be described as physiological, and was not due to bone destruction in which citrate has been

implicated. One can conclude from the literature that while vitamin D almost certainly has a direct effect on citrate metabolism in bone, this seems to have little connection with the calcification mechanism, but the levels of blood and bone citrate seem to have some correlation. A good deal of citrate exists passively in bone, complexed with the apatite crystal (Armstrong and Singer, 1965), and some must participate in the tricarboxylic acid cycle. Vitamin D has effects upon other tissues besides bone. For example, DeLuca and Steenbock (1957) found it to suppress the oxidation of citrate and isocitrate by the kidney mitochondria of both normal and rachitic rats, and Mendelsohn (1962) found that the addition of vitamin D to the reaction mixture of oral tissue from rachitic rats restored the activation of ATPase by dinitrophenol, which did not occur in the absence of the vitamin. Vitamin D appears to be concerned with the metabolism of a number of different tissues, one of which is bone.

Chapter 11

ACTION OF ENDOCRINE GLANDS ON BONE AND CALCIUM AND PHOSPHORUS METABOLISM

Hypophysis

As is well known, this gland regulates bone growth; this is seen clinically during its overactivity in such conditions as acromegaly and gigantism. The earlier work of Becks and his group showed that after hypophysectomy all growth sequences in endochondral bone formation stopped (Becks *et al.*, 1945). Using the recently available growth hormone, they reported that when this was administered to normal animals, the growth sequences persisted and the bones were larger and longer (Evans *et al.*, 1948). When given to hypophysectomized animals, endochondral bone formation was at once stimulated (Kibrick *et al.*, 1941) and persisted as long as the hormone was given. Closure of epiphyses was only attained if thyroxine was given as well (Simpson *et al.*, 1944). Within recent years, human growth hormone has become available in limited amounts, and is being used in the treatment of clinical conditions, since bovine hormone is not active in humans. This has stimulated fresh work in this field. Thus Harris and Heaney (1969) found in dogs that growth hormone increased the skeletal mass and bone apposition. The accretion rate was increased, endosteal resorption was inhibited, and extensive endosteal new bone was formed. As stated elsewhere, this approach is of interest in the treatment of osteoporosis.

The similarity in appearance of bone in inanition and after hypophysectomy has led to the supposition that in inanition the growth hormone is withdrawn (Acheson, 1959). Irving (1956b), however, has pointed out that while hypophysectomy caused extensive changes in the rat's continually erupting incisor tooth, protein deficiency had no such effect and that the similarity of appearances in the two conditions was only coincidental.

The effect of growth hormone on bone does not seem to be a direct one. Rigal (1964) found that explanted bone from rabbits given the hormone before the bone was removed showed an increase in the mitotic activity of the cells of the growth plate, but this effect could not be duplicated by adding growth hormone to the medium.

Cortisone

The action of this hormone in general is to retard or suppress the activity of the growth plate, but the effect seems to be species dependent (Follis, 1951). Thus, in rats, the epiphyseal cartilage is diminished in width and calcified cartilage is retained in the trabeculae of the primary spongiosa (Laron and Boss, 1962; Hulth and Olerud, 1963), while in the rabbit a bony plate seals off the metaphysis (Storey, 1958). Chick embryo bone formation is retarded (Siegel et al., 1957). Laron et al. (1858a,b) found that on a low calcium diet the width of growth plate of rats, which diminished while on this regime, was further reduced by cortisone, and that the calcemic effect of parathyroid hormone was abolished. Although cortisone given in unphysiological amounts has the effects described above, it probably has little specific effect upon bone formation other than its well-known general antianabolic action.

Estrogens

The action of estrogens on bone is of great interest. It was first noted by Kyes and Potter in 1934 that the female pigeon during the egg-laying period developed an excess of spongy bone in the marrow cavity of the long bone (medullary bone). When the calcium was needed for eggshell formation the excess bone was rapidly removed. During this time, from preovulation till the eggs were laid, the blood calcium rose to high figures. Male hormones had no such effect and the removal of the hypophysis or parathyroids did not prevent the hypercalcaemia (Riddle and McDonald, 1945). The effect on bone could be reproduced in male pigeons and also in mice (female and male) by the administration of estrogen (Gardner and Pfeiffer, 1939). The local application of estradiol to chips of bone implanted in the brain of littermate mice was not followed by any bone change (Barnicot, 1951).

Urist (1967) reported that when parathyroid hormone was given to laying hens, resorption was only seen in endosteal bone. Intramedullary bone was unchanged and could be affected only by estrogen. Simmons (1966) considered that the effect of estrogen was to stimulate the differentiation of osteoblasts, but the ability of individual osteoblasts to synthesize and form collagen was unchanged.

The levels of blood calcium, phosphorus, and phosphatase of mice do not change when estrogens are given. Urist *et al.* (1948) investigated the action of estrogens in other animals, and of those they tested found young rats the only ones to be affected, but in a rather different way. Here the resorption of cartilage and new bone was prevented so that a very large spongiosa developed. Simkiss (1961) found that no medullary bone formation occurred in turtles or tortoises after administration of estrogen, and Suzuki and Prosser (1968) reported that while blood calcium and phosphorus changes were caused in a lizard, no medullary bone formation occurred.

The principal effect of estrogens in bone formation is concerned with egg-laying in birds, and the reason for a somewhat similar action in some mammals is not very evident as it appears to fulfil no physiological need. In pregnant mice neither the fetal nor maternal skeletons show any medullary bone formation.

The Parathyroid Gland

This is the most important endocrine as regards calcium metabolism, since its hormone, together with calcitonin, produced by ultimobranchial cells or their derivatives, controls calcium homeostasis in the body.

Gley (1893) first recognized that the tetany sometimes seen after thyroidectomy was due to concurrent removal of the parathyroids, but it was not till 1923 that Salvesen established the relation between hypocalcemia and tetany in hypoparathyroidism. The relationship between parathyroid tumors and von Recklinghausen's disease of bone was recognized in 1930 (Bauer et al., 1930).

Since the preparation of an active extract in 1926 by Collip, it has been possible to study in detail the mechanism of its action, which is twofold, on bone, controlling resorption, and on the renal tubule, regulating phosphate reabsorption. For a while it was considered that the renal tubular effect was the primary one (Albright and Ellsworth, 1929) but it is now known that the hormone has two primary effects; this has recently been confirmed by the elegant experiments on the intervention of cyclic AMP in parathyroid hormone action.

Keutmann et al. (1971) have isolated the predominant form of the hormone from bovine parathyroid glands, as well as two other biologically active peptides. All three contained 84 amino acid residues, had alanine as the amino terminal acid, and did not contain cystine. The calculated molecular weight of the predominant hormone was 9563. The same group (Woodhead et al., 1971) have prepared porcine parathyroid hormone, which differed in some respects from bovine in its amino acid composition, serine being the amino terminal acid. The calculated molecular weight was 9423. Interesting results on the structural requirements for biological activity were reported.

Hargis et al. (1964) and Perkin et al. (1968), using immunofluorescent techniques, have shown that the hormone is located in the chief cells of the gland and between cords of acini, but not in the oxyphil cells. Buckle (1969) stated that the half life of parathyroid hormone in the body was 20 minutes and that complete resynthesis in the gland could occur as frequently as once every 30 minutes. It was thus possible that variations in hormone secretion could exercise a more important role in the minute-by-minute regulation of calcium homeostasis than commonly recognised.

The action of the hormone on bone is possibly twofold. It initially increases lysozomal enzymes and later increases osteoclast production. Toto and Magon (1966) found after one injection of parathyroid hormone that labeled osteoclasts appeared 12 hours later, and had disappeared between 48 and 72 hours after injection. Toft and Talmage

(1960) developed an osteoclast-counting method that could be used as an index of parathyroid gland activity. The direct effect of parathyroid hormone on osteoclast production had been earlier described by Barnicot (1948) and Chang (1951) as occurring when fragments of bone and parathyroid gland were grafted together either intracerebrally or subperiosteally. Parathyroid hormone can also act *in vitro*. Gaillard (1959) demonstrated that both parathyroid glands or parathyroid extract incubated with mouse embryo bone caused bone resorption, and Raisz (1963a) reported the same, but pointed out that the bone must be alive for resorption to occur. Stern *et al.* (1963) labeled the collagen of fetal calvaria and found the liberation of proline and hydroxyproline into the medium to be accelerated by parathyroid hormone, a true digestion occurring. The same has been shown *in vivo* (Bates *et al.*, 1964). Avioli and Prokop (1967) reported, working with rhesus monkeys, that parathyroid extract could cause the degradation of insoluble bone collagen and possibly also that of soluble collagen. Walker *et al.* (1964) had previously put epiphyseal cartilages on to collagen gels and studied the digestion of the collagen. This was markedly increased with bone from parathyroid-treated animals, the optimal effects being seen in bones taken 36 hours after hormone injection. Bélanger and Migicovsky (1963), using a similar technique, found that parathyroid hormone increased the collagenolytic activity of osteocytes.

It is also possible that osteoblast activity in bone is retarded by parathyroid hormone. This has been suggested by Dawson *et al.* (1957), and Flanagan and Nichols (1969) found parathyroid hormone to diminish collagen synthesis in bone *in vitro*. Heller-Steinberg (1951) had earlier noted that the hormone had an action of the polymerization of the ground substance of bone. Several workers have reported that the hormone causes an increased turnover of glycosaminoglycans (Bernstein and Handler, 1958; Johnson *et al.*, 1962; Guri and Bernstein, 1964). Johnston *et al.* (1965) considered the action to be direct on bone and irrespective of calcium ion changes. These effects may well be carried out by osteocytes, especially since Bélanger and Robichon (1964) found that parathyroid hormone acts on these cells causing osteolysis. In view of the findings mentioned below of the speed with which parathyroid hormone can be released, it is conceivable that its first action is on osteocytes.

As far as calcium removal is concerned, it seems that both recently laid-down and also older calcium can be resorbed. Bronner (1957) found the most recently laid-down calcium to be removed while Woods and Armstrong (1956) reported that calcium incarcerated in the stable bone mineral could also be mobilized. Clark and Geoffroy (1958) confirmed both these findings, radiocalcium given 2 days before dosage, or 60 days before, being equally well acted on. Richelle and Bronner (1963) reported that the percentage of exchangeable calcium was increased by parathyroid hormone, an alteration in the ultrastructural relationships between organic and mineral phases occurring before resorption. Jeffay and Boyne (1964) determined more exactly which bone calcium was mobilized, finding that about one quarter came from a slowly exchanging fraction of bone, and three quarters from recently apposed or labeled bone. It is easy to visualize the removal of recently laid down calcium, but the mobilization of calcium from the stable bone mineral must involve some change in the organic matrix as suggested by Heller-Steinberg and Richelle and Bronner, which makes the calcium in these areas more available. Conversely, Raisz and Hammack (1959) found after parathyroidectomy, that there was a decrease in the "six-hour exchangeable calcium." This they attributed to a decreased bone resorption, leading to decreased bone apposition, and thus less available calcium.

CONTROL OF PARATHYROID HORMONE SECRETION

The blood calcium level is the sole factor controlling parathyroid hormone secretion. Raisz et al. (1965) found that hypophysectomy did not affect the metabolism or size of the parathyroids, nor did growth hormone; thus the requirement for parathyroid hormone was not related to new bone formation or bone turnover. Roth et al. (1968) reported that, provided the serum calcium was unaltered, a variety of parameters, including changes in serum inorganic phosphorus, calcium:phosphate ratio of serum or diet, or presence or absence of vitamin D had no effect on parathyroid gland activity.

The factors controlling parathyroid hormone secretion have been studied in a variety of ways. The size of the gland has been used as a criterion. Stoerck and Carnes showed in 1945 that there was an inverse relationship between the gland size and the blood calcium level. This has been often confirmed since then (e.g., G. A. Williams *et al.*, 1964; Au and Raisz, 1965). The metabolism of the parathyroids has also been taken as an index of gland activity. Pearse and Tremblay (1958) studied the level of leucine aminopeptidase in the gland and reported the amount of this enzyme to be reduced by a large dose of dihydrotachysterol and increased by low calcium diets, there being a correlation between the enzyme activity and hormone production. Cheeseman *et al.* (1964) reported similarly that vitamin D deficiency caused an increase of leucine aminopeptidase in the parathyroid. The α-aminoisobutyric acid uptake has been studied *in vitro* and *in vivo* by several groups. Increasing the calcium in the medium of the incubated gland depressed the uptake of this amino acid, an effect not seen with a variety of other hormones or obtained with other glands (Raisz and O'Brien, 1963). G. A. Williams *et al.* (1964) and Au and Raisz (1965) reported similar findings *in vivo*. Raisz (1967) incubated parathyroid glands in media containing a number of amino acids, and found the uptake of these to be greater in low compared to high calcium-containing solutions. This effect was a direct one on amino acid uptake, since it was not affected by puromycin, actinomycin D, or ouabain.

Several workers have reported results in which the parathyroid hormone level in blood has been estimated, usually by immunoassay methods. The release of parathyroid hormone had a reciprocal relationship to the blood calcium ion level. Several papers comment on the speed with which parathyroid hormone is released (e.g., Copp and Davidson, 1961; Care *et al.*, 1966) when the blood calcium is lowered. Parathyroid glands cultivated *in vitro* also released the hormone when the calcium content of the medium was lowered (Raisz, 1963b).

Many of these findings were anticipated by McLean and Urist (1955) when they postulated that a negative feedback mechanism regulated the production of parathyroid hormone, the blood calcium ion level being the stimulus to which the gland responded. After parathyroidectomy, the blood calcium sinks to a value of about 1.75 mM, and this level is maintained by a chemical equilibrium with labile bone mineral. The difference between the normal level, 2.5 mM, and this lower figure is maintained by the parathyroid gland by this feedback mechanism. This concept has been modified to some extent by the discovery of the action of calcitonin, but in essence remains the same as when first enunciated.

Long-standing hypercalcemia in dogs did not affect the histology of the parathyroid glands, nor was any sign of atrophy found (Schmidt *et al.*, 1966).

EFFECT ON THE BLOOD CALCIUM LEVEL

The injection of parathyroid hormone causes a hypercalcemia, the speed of which depends upon the purity of the preparation. Rasmussen and Westall (1956) found that crude extracts caused a maximal hypercalcemia at 18 hours, but their purified extract produced a maximal hypercalcemia at 6 hours, the calcium level returning to normal at 18 hours. Breen and Freeman (1961) studied the effect of the hormone on the various fractions of blood calcium in rats and dogs. Normal and hypercalcemic animals had a relatively higher proportion of diffusible calcium than hypocalcemic ones. The binding of calcium rose as the total calcium rose, but did not follow the law of mass action as usually expressed. Calcium added to hypocalcemic blood had the same distribution as that in animals injected with parathyroid hormone.

After parathyroidectomy the blood calcium falls and the condition of tetany occurs when the calcium level is about 1.25 mM. This condition is characterized by increased sensitivity of the neuromuscular junction and leads to typical muscle spasms, although it has been suggested by Greenberg *et al.* (1942) that a part of the central nervous system higher than the spinal cord is involved.

RENAL ACTION OF THE PARATHYROID

The other action of parathyroid hormone is on phosphate reabsorption by the tubules of the kidney. Samiy *et al.* (1960, 1965), using their stop flow technique on parathyroidectomized dogs, showed quite clearly that the hormone caused a marked increase in phosphate excretion and a significant fall in phosphate reabsorption. There was no increase in the filtered load and probably both proximal and distal segments of the nephron were affected, although the proximal did most of the reabsorbing. They got no evidence that parathyroid hormone mediated a secretory process for phosphate excretion. Mayer *et al.* (1966) also reported that in cows the phosphaturia caused by the hormone was due almost entirely to a depression of tubular reabsorption of phosphate. Hiatt and Thompson (1957) found that an acute dose of parathyroid hormone in humans caused phosphaturia by altering renal hemodynamics and without an accompanying hypercalcemia, but prolonged administration decreased T_m for phosphate and caused a hypercalcemia. An even earlier effect was reported by Hellman *et al.* (1965) working with parathyroidectomized dogs and with humans. This was that before a rise in phosphate excretion had occurred, an inhibition of sodium ion for hydrogen ion exchange took place, possibly by interfering directly with the ability of the kidney to maintain a hydrogen ion concentration gradient between body fluids and the tubular urine. Foulks (1956) and Foulks and Perry (1959) thought that the rapid phosphaturia after injection of phosphate was not due to parathyroid action but, as indicated above, the parathyroids can secrete their hormone very rapidly.

Eisenberg (1965) has pointed out that a phosphate homeostatic mechanism can exist independent of the parathyroid glands, since hypoparathyroid patients could excrete phosphate quite normally when infused with calcium. Thus it is possible that the calcium level of the blood may play a role in the action of the parathyroids on renal phosphate excretion.

The findings on the influence of the hormone on renal calcium excretion are conflicting and possible species dependent. Bacon *et al.* (1956) found parathyroid hormone to increase calcium excretion in the urine of rats, while Buchanan *et al.* (1959) found a decrease in urinary calcium in mice. Walser (1969), in a review article on the subject, concluded that there was a high calcium clearance in relation to plasma calcium in parathyroid insufficiency, and the opposite effect after administration of parathyroid hormone, the site of action being distal.

The two effects of the hormone can be separated by actinomycin D. Eisenstein and Passavoy (1964) reported that this compound prevented the hypercalcemia and inhibited bone changes (it also inhibited the bone changes caused by large doses of vitamin D). Rasmussen *et al.* (1964) found the same but the usual renal action was not affected. Both groups commented that the action of actinomycin D might be by inhibiting the synthesis of proteins or enzymes which degraded bone. Raisz (1965) studied embryo bone *in vitro* and reported that actinomycin D inhibited cell proliferation and prevented the bone resorption caused by parathyroid hormone. With small amounts of actinomycin D, parathyroid hormone could overcome the actinomycin D effect, and thus might act competitively.

Reaven *et al.* (1959) noted that parathyroid hormone *in vitro* inhibited the uptake of labeled calcium by voluntary muscle and suggested that the hormone could regulate calcium movement between extra- and intracellular fluid. A similar suggestion was made by Borle 1968). Mears (1969) proposed that both parathyroid hormone and calcitonin could act on an osteogenic cell membrane calcium pump which controlled the rate of RNA synthesis and ultimately protein synthesis. Foulks and Perry (1959) considered that parathyroid hormone could also regulate the transfer of phosphate out of the extracellular fluid compartment. It is possible that the action of parathyroid hormone is much wider than has been considered heretofore. Thus Cohn *et al.* (1967) found that it caused the accumulation of calcium and phosphate ions in kidney mitochondria and Rasmussen *et al.* (1967), working with liver and kidney mitochondria, reported that parathyroid hormone stimulated decarboxylation of a variety of Krebs cycle intermediates, the effect being highly specific to the hormone and closely correlated with its hypercalcemic activity. Nitrated hormone, which is less hypercalcemic, had a lesser effect. Norman (1967), however, feels that it is probably too early to be able to state that these actions on mitochondria are a valid measure of the *in vivo* physiological action of the hormone. Thus parathyroid hormone is not known to have any action on the liver in the intact animal; possibly the results are more chemical interactions than physiologically significant effects. However, the information gained on membrane phenomena is of great general importance.

The effects of parathyroid hormone on bone metabolism have also been studied. Cohn and Forscher (1962) gave rabbits the hormone and investigated the enzyme activity of their tissues. Bone and kidney, but not liver or muscle, produced more CO_2 than the controls, probably of Krebs cycle origin, derived from glucose. They thought the increased hydrogen ion production could shift the relative proportions of ionic forms of phosphate, possibly influencing phosphate reabsorption in the kidney and certainly increasing the rate of dissolution of bone mineral. Much of the biochemical evidence suggests that parathyroid hormone increases citrate production in bone. Hekkelman (1961) found the level of isocitric dehydrogenase in bone to be decreased by parathyroid hormone. Lekan *et al.* (1960) found that parathyroid hormone pretreatment caused a greatly increased production of citrate from labeled pyruvate by bone *in vitro*. In similar experiments, Chattopadhyay and Freeman (1965) pretreated animals with the hormone and then incubated the bone with labeled glucose. Much more citrate (and malate) were produced, compared with controls, but lactate production was little influenced. On the other hand, Borle *et al.* (1960) found that lactate was produced in much larger amounts after pretreatment with parathyroid hormone, citrate being hardly affected. Cohn and Forscher (1961) had no evidence that citrate metabolism was affected by the hormone. Herrmann-Eilee (1964) investigated the lactic dehydrogenase activity of epiphyseal and hypertrophic cartilage of embryonic mouse bone, and found it to be reduced by parathyroid hormone. This contradictory evidence must be largely caused by the different techniques used. It is a pity that these workers could not all get together and do a conjoint experiment, which might possibly settle their differences. In any case, the present author, as stated above, personally favors the citrate hypothesis.

INTESTINAL ACTION OF THE PARATHYROID

There is some evidence that parathyroid hormone may influence the absorption of calcium or phosphate in the gut. Borle *et al.* (1963) produced results with perfused everted gut sacs that parathyroid hormone could increase phosphate absorption. As far as calcium is concerned, Winter *et al.* (1970) reported that absorption was decreased in rats by parathyroidectomy and Payne and Sansom (1966) found the same in goats. However, Mayer *et al.* (1967), working with cows, found that parathyroid hormone produced a decrease in intestinal calcium absorption. In 1968, they reported that fecal phosphorus was decreased in cows by parathyroid extract, but did not commit themselves as to whether the hormone controlled phosphorus absorption. Sammon *et al.* (1970) found that parathyroid hormone had no effect on intestinal absorption of calcium or phosphorus. It is generally felt that if the hormone does control intestinal absorption of calcium or phosphate, this is a minor action compared with its effects on bone and kidney.

Vitamin D and Parathyroid Action

In 1958 Harrison *et al.* reported that parathyroid hormone had no action on vitamin D-deficient rats. This dependence of the hormone action on the concomitant presence of vitamin D has not been confirmed by some other workers (Toverud, 1964; Au and Raisz, 1965; Nichols *et al.*, 1963) working with both *in vivo* and *in vitro* systems. Arnaud *et al.* (1966) reported that vitamin D was necessary for the mobilization of calcium and phosphate from bone by parathyroid hormone, but not for its phosphaturic action. Hurwitz *et al.* (1969) found that the blood calcium could not be maintained in the animals on a diet deficient in vitamin D but otherwise normal, suggesting that the vitamin was necessary for calcium mobilization by the parathyroids. It is rather hard to come to a definite conclusion as to the relationship between the hormone and the vitamin. At the most, vitamin D may be essential only for bone resorption by parathyroid hormone. Vitamin D in large doses does have a bone resorptive action and it may be that the two agents act synergistically. They probably act through a similar mechanism, since, as stated above, the bone resorptive action of both is inhibited by actinomycin D.

Cyclic AMP

In 1958 Sutherland and Rall described a cyclic nucleotide which accumulated in the liver as a result of epinephrine administration. Since then, this compound, cyclic AMP (adenosine 3′,5′-monophosphate) has been implicated as an intermediate in the action of many peptide hormones and in the release of neurotransmitters at synapses and neuromuscular junctions. It was also found that its action was closely bound up with the calcium ion. A review of this subject has recently been published (H. Rasmussen, 1970).

Cyclic AMP is synthesized by adenyl cyclase from adenosine triphosphate in the presence of magnesium ions. The enzyme is associated with cell membranes. Cyclic AMP is broken down by a relatively specific phosphodiesterase, this enzyme being inhibited by theophylline. From the existing data, the idea has emerged that cyclic AMP is the second messenger, the first messenger being an external stimulus specific for the particular cell type. This first messenger interacts with membrane-bound adenyl cyclase causing increased cyclic AMP synthesis within the cell, which as second messenger activates one or more processes or enzymes. An enormous number of processes controlled by these reactions have been described, and it may well be queried as to how such a wide range of actions can be specific in any particular case. It is probable that the specificity resides in the hormone which is acting, as well as in the cell on which it acts.

CYCLIC AMP AND THE PARATHYROID HORMONE

As far as the parathyroid gland is concerned there is growing evidence that its hormone also acts through the cyclic AMP mechanism. Vaes (1968a) used the dibutyryl derivative, which is more stable than cyclic AMP, and found that dibutyryl cyclic AMP acted on bone cultures in a similar way to parathyroid hormone and was hypercalcemic in parathyroidectomized rats; the latter action has also been described by Wells and Lloyd (1967, 1969). Rasmussen *et al.* (1968) also reported that cyclic AMP mimicked all the actions of parathyroid hormone in parathyroidectomized rats, the mobilization of calcium and hydroxyproline from bone being blocked by calcitonin. Herrmann-Eilee and Konijn (1970), using embryonic mouse calvaria, reported that parathyroid hormone increased the cyclic AMP content.

Nagata and Rasmussen (1968) found that parathyroid hormone caused an increase in renal cell cyclic AMP in normal and vitamin D-deficient animals, and the same was found in a renal cell suspension from normal animals by Michelakis (1970). Douša and Rychlík (1968) used kidney homogenates and found that parathyroid hormone caused an increase in adenyl cyclase production, the effect being dose dependant. Agus *et al.* (1971) have reported the same.

Probably the most quantitative experiments have been carried out by Aurbach and Chase. Their work has been recently summarized (1970). Parathyroid hormone injected into parathyroidectomized rats within minutes caused a sharp rise in the rate of cyclic AMP excretion in the urine, this event preceding the rise in phosphate elimination. They showed that parathyroid hormone when added to homogenates of kidney tissue caused a fivefold increase in activation of adenyl cyclase, which was detected within 15 seconds of adding the hormone to the enzyme preparation. Incidentally, as would be expected, adenyl cyclase was found primarily associated with the plasma membrane fractions. Later experiments showed the enzyme to be located in the tubular elements of the renal cortex.

Aurbach and Chase then investigated bone, using homogenized fragments of rat fetal calvaria, and found that enzyme activity was greatly increased by parathyroid hormone, being a direct function of the logarithm of the hormone concentration. This phenomenon was strictly specific for parathyroid hormone; conversely, parathyroid hormone did not affect the adenyl cyclase activity in a number of other tissues tested. Unexpectedly, fluoride was a powerful activator of adenyl cyclase. Calcitonin, although it inhibits bone resorption and the hypercalcemic effect of parathyroid hormone or dibutyryl cyclic AMP, did not prevent the basal activity of adenyl cyclase or the stimulating effect of parathyroid hormone, and thus must act on same step subsequent to the formation of cyclic AMP. But, strangely enough, calcitonin has been reported to stimulate the formation of cyclic AMP in both kidney and bone preparations (Murad *et al.*, 1970).

Prostaglandins have been postulated to interact in several hormonal systems. Beck *et al.* (1970) have reported that prostaglandin E_1 inhibited, in an *in vitro* system, the increase in adenyl cyclase and in cyclic AMP caused by parathyroid hormone in renal tissue. After renal artery injection in dogs, it also inhibited the parathyroid hormone-induced increase in urinary phosphate excretion. The evidence they adduced suggested that this substance acted by inhibiting adenyl cyclase activity.

As stated elsewhere, it is still not completely proved that parathyroid hormone acts in the intestine. However, Harrison and Harrison (1970) have claimed that the hormone has such an action, and that cyclic AMP is involved. Both activities require the presence of vitamin D.

The evidence cited above shows that parathyroid hormone acts on the two main target organs, bone and the kidneys, through the adenyl cyclase–cyclic AMP system, and that the activation of adenyl cyclase is the true primary effect of the hormone. Thus a single mechanism can

explain its action on two diverse tissues and the cyclic AMP thus formed intracellularly activates processes according to the various physiological effects of parathyroid hormone.

Calcitonin

In 1962 Copp and Cameron reported the existence of a new hormone
which had a quick hypocalcemic action. They found this factor in com-
mercial preparations of parathyroid hormone, the hypocalcemic
action being followed shortly after by the hypercalcemic effect. On
perfusing the parathyroid gland with a high calcium solution, Copp and
Cheyney (1962) reported that there was a dramatic fall in the systemic
blood calcium, a fast-acting effect and short-lived. They called the new
factor calcitonin.

Subsequent work showed that in almost all mammals the thyroid
gland was the source of this hormone, only human parathyroid also
containing calcitonin (Galante *et al.*, 1968) Hirsch *et al.* (1963) made
a crude extract of thyroid which was rich in calcitonin, and in order to
avoid confusion they called this hormone thyrocalcitonin. However,
subsequent work has shown that this name is not necessary, and most
workers call the hypocalcemic factor calcitonin.

Perfusion experiments were complicated by the fact that the thyroid
and parathyroid share the same circulation in many animals. However,
the goat has a parathyroid gland with a separate blood supply, and
advantage was taken of this by Foster *et al.* (1964). They found that
perfusion of this gland alone with a high calcium solution did not cause
the release of calcitonin. The thyroid gland had to be in the circuit for
the effect to be obtained. This has been confirmed by a number of
workers.

After showing that the thyroid was the main and probably the only
source of calcitonin in most mammals, a search was undertaken for the
cells involved. Bussolati and Pearse (1967), using immunofluorescent
methods, found that calcitonin was localized in the C cells (sometimes
called clear, or parafollicular cells). Capen and Young (1969), working
with cows, reported that large doses of vitamin D caused a decrease
in granule content and hypertrophy of the parafollicular cells. After
vitamin D dosage ceased, the cells returned to a resting state, but the

calcitonin response was unable to prevent the hypercalcemia caused by vitamin D.

A considerable advance occurred when Copp *et al.* (1967) found that the ultimobranchial bodies of sharks and fowls contained a great deal of calcitonin. These bodies arise from the last branchial pouch in elasmobranchs, bony fish, amphibia, reptiles, birds, and mammals, fish having no parathyroid glands. The ultimobranchial bodies are separate entities in all genera except mammals, and in the latter types they are embedded in the thyroid gland as parafollicular cells. Moseley *et al.* (1968) confirmed the findings of Copp *et al.*, and this discovery has given the ultimobranchial apparatus an endocrine role, and has identified biochemically the origin of the parafollicular cells of the thyroid.

COMPOSITION OF CALCITONINS

So far, the bovine, porcine, salmon, and human calcitonins have been isolated and identified. They are all peptides, containing 32 amino acids. Porcine calcitonin has two forms of equal potency, one containing methionine as the sulfoxide, the other in the reduced form (Brewer *et al.*, 1968). Human calcitonin differs somewhat from porcine in having no arginine or tryptophan, but containing lysine and isoleucine, absent in the porcine form (Byfield *et al.*, 1969). In a later paper Brewer *et al.* (1970) analyzed bovine calcitonin and reported that it differed from the other calcitonins in some amino residues. All forms agreed in having the carboxyl terminal amino acid as prolinamide. The molecular weight of calcitonin is about 3500. For some reason salmon calcitonin is much more potent than porcine in rats and rabbits (Copp, 1969). A unit of potency has been established by the British Medical Research Council based on the fall in plasma calcium. Brewer *et al.* (1968, 1970) reported porcine and bovine calcitonin to have a potency of 200 units/mg and Byfield *et al.* (1969) found the human hormone to have 135 units/mg. Salmon calcitonin is about 25 times as potent.

ACTION OF CALCITONIN

Calcitonin causes hypocalcemia, hypophosphatemia, and phosphaturia (Kenny and Heiskell, 1965; Milhaud and Moukhtar, 1966). Kenny and Heiskell stated that neither the kidney nor the gut played any role in the hypocalcemic response. The above findings have been confirmed in general by most workers, but there are some species differences. Thus it has been reported that porcine calcitonin lowers the serum calcium in monkeys and man, but has no effect on serum phosphate (Bell *et al.*, 1966). When porcine calcitonin was given to dogs there was no change in renal calcium excretion (Clark *et al.*, 1968), whereas Ardaillou *et al.* (1969) considered that porcine calcitonin could increase both calcium and phosphate excretion in man. Aldred *et al.* (1970) gave rats salmon calcitonin and found in addition to hypocalcemia, an increase in urinary calcium and phosphate. Porcine calcitonin produced only the blood changes. Probably the true effect of calcitonin will only be known when it is injected into an animal of the same species from which it was isolated.

The blood calcium level affects the response to calcitonin. If the blood calcium is abnormally low, calcitonin has no effect (Bell and Stern, 1970). However, Morii and DeLuca (1967) found that calcitonin would lower the blood calcium of vitamin D-deficient rats, when parathyroid hormone had no effect upon the blood calcium level.

The fundamental action of calcitonin is to inhibit bone resorption. This has been unequivocally demonstrated by many workers both *in vivo* and *in vitro*. Aliapoulios *et al.* (1966), using the Goldhaber bone culture system, found the bone resorption caused by parathyroid hormone to be inhibited, as well as that caused by vitamin A, calcitonin thus acting on a basic site of bone resorption. Reynolds and Dingle (1970) also reported, using labeled calvaria in organ culture, that calcitonin inhibited the formation of new osteoclasts and the action of those already present, when stimulated by either parathyroid hormone or vitamin A in the medium. Friedman and Raisz (1965), also working *in vitro*, found osteoclast proliferation caused by parathyroid hormone to be inhibited. They considered that calcitonin did not compete with parathyroid hormone for a single site of action, but acted at a different site of the mechanism of bone resorption. Klein and Talmage (1968) found that extracellular hydroxyproline was reduced as was the release of calcium, so that calcitonin inhibited the entire process of bone catabolism. However, the anabolic aspect of bone was unchanged; Flanagan and Nichols (1969) reported that calcitonin did not affect collagen synthesis *in vitro*. The action on bone is greatly reduced in older animals (Copp and Kuczerpa, 1968) which is to be expected since bone turnover rate is reduced with age.

Soft tissue calcification and calciphylactic calcification of skin were found to be prevented by calcitonin (Gabbiani *et al.*, 1968). The hypocalcemia caused by glucagon has been shown to be due to the release of calcitonin (Avioli *et al.*, 1969a).

It may finally be asked what part, if any, calcitonin plays in calcium homeostasis. Brown *et al.* (1969) removed all ultimobranchial tissues from chicks and found no change in the blood calcium, phosphorus, or alkaline phosphatase of bone. They concluded that calcitonin had no major role in skeletal growth, but that the fall in blood calcium after hypercalcemia caused by parathyroid hormone was calcitonin dependent. Sammon *et al.* (1969) gave calcitonin to parathyroidectomized rats with different levels of calcium intake. No effect was seen on net calcium absorption in the intestine, net calcium balance in bone, or on urinary excretion or kidney function in regulating plasma calcium. Calcitonin had no steady-state effect on calcium metabolism or homeostasis in contrast to the parathyroid glands, interruption of whose function caused a significant decrease in the regulation of calcium metabolism. On the other hand, Munson and Gray (1969) gave a "modest" amount of calcium by stomach tube to intact, fasted rats, and got little or no hypercalcemia, but rats acutely thyroidectomized had hypercalcemia.

One is thus left in the position that only future work can decide on the physiological role of this hormone. The present writer has always thought that the problem of blood calcium regulation was to maintain it at normal levels, not to lower it. Conceivably calcitonin may come into action when the blood calcium rises to dangerously high levels, but it is not always effective in this regard, at least under experimental conditions.

Thyroid

Thyroidectomy causes a slowing in the rate of bone growth and differentiation. Endochondral ossification goes on, but at a very slow rate, so that the bone of a 72-day-old rat has the appearance of that of one 15–20 days old. As mentioned above, growth hormone stimulates growth but not differentiation of the tissues of the thyroidectomized animal, whereas if thyroxine is given, both growth and differentiation occur (Becks *et al.*, 1950). Long-continued overactivity of the gland produces osteoporosis, and the administration of the extract to normal animals causes an increased calcium excretion (Albright *et al.*, 1931). The increased fecal excretion is due to a diminution of both passive and active calcium transport (Noble and Matty, 1967).

Thyroxine increases the bone turnover rate in rats (Milhaud, 1965) and the same has been found in humans. Krane *et al.* (1956) found in patients with hyperthyroidism that the pool size of exchangeable calcium increased, with a considerable increase in bone calcium turnover, whereas in hypothyroidism Heaney and Whedon (1958) reported that the decreased bone calcium turnover rate could be increased by giving thyroid extract. Care (1968) has pointed out, on the basis of these findings, that there may be a physiological interaction between this hormone and calcitonin, which inhibits bone resorption.

Osteoporosis

This phenomenon can be regarded as an exaggeration of a process that apparently normally happens after middle age. Only when clinical symptoms such as backache and vertebral fractures occur, can osteoporosis be said to have begun. The condition is apparently due to excessive bone resorption compared to apposition.

Garn *et al.* (1967) have surveyed bone loss in men and women in the United States, Guatemala, and El Salvador, using a radiogrammetric measurement of cortical bone in the hand skeleton. They found that in all three countries bone loss began in the fifth decade, and progressed much more rapidly in women than in men. Their results agreed with those of Nordin's W.H.O. survey (1964).

In an endeavor to find out the cause of this "normal" bone loss, and also a reason for osteoporosis, many investigations have been undertaken and hypotheses invoked. Since postmenopausal osteoporosis is common in women, Albright *et al.* (1940) suggested that the disease had an endocrine basis. He claimed (1947) to get good results with estrogen therapy, but the balance of results since then have shown this treatment to be disappointing. Another hypothesis that has been advanced is that a long-standing calcium deficiency is the cause. Many years ago Owen *et al.* (1939) reported that osteoporotic males, who had been on a low calcium intake for some time, could store calcium if the intake was raised. Similar findings were reported by Nicolaysen *et al.* (1953) and many others, and Vinther-Paulsen (1953) considered that the incidence of senile osteoporosis was related to the level of calcium intake.

More recently Nordin (1962) and Dallas and Nordin (1962) have suggested that a chronic low calcium intake (due to an inability to adapt to an inadequate intake or to a higher than normal calcium requirement) might be the cause of osteoporosis. Dallas and Nordin pointed out that a negative balance of 100 mg Ca/day would involve the removal of 36.5 g from the skeleton each year. If clinical osteoporosis involved the destruction of approximately 30% of the skeleton, this could be accomplished in 10 years, and thus the disease would become more frequent with advancing age, which in fact is usually the case. Spencer *et al.* (1964) have found that certain patients with osteoporosis have a defect in calcium absorption and Hurxthal and Vose (1969) produced clinical evidence that the calcium intake over a period of years was one of the factors in the causation of osteoporosis. Bullamore *et al.* (1970) reported that the level of intestinal calcium absorption fell with age after about 60 years and all their subjects over 80 had significant malabsorption. They followed the level of radiocalcium in the plasma after oral administration, and thought that a relative vitamin D deficiency might be a possible cause. Cohn *et al.* (1968) found, using kinetic methods with 7 osteoporotic patients, that 2.5 g of calcium/day caused a decrease in the resorption rate of bone, apposition being only slightly affected.

However, Garn *et al.* (1967) produced evidence that the level of the calcium intake was not a significant factor in the incidence of osteoporosis. They studied 400 persons on a long-term longitudinal basis, analyzing their diets and following the course of bone change. Absolutely no correlation was found between calcium intake and bone loss. Smith and Frame (1965) and Exton-Smith *et al.* (1966) had also found no correlation between calcium intake and bone density. Shah *et al.* (1967), working with aged mice, likewise found that the porosity of the bones was not related to the calcium content of the diet.

Other suggestions for the cause of the condition have been made. Thus Wachman and Bernstein (1968) thought that the "acid ash" type of diet usually consumed by humans could be causative. One mEq of fixed acid would require for neutralization 2 mEq of calcium, causing a 15% loss of the skeleton over 10 years. It would be interesting to know why dogs, eating a very acid diet, do not suffer more from osteoporosis.

Birge *et al.* (1967) reported an association between osteoporosis and primary lactose deficiency. Lactose has been considered by some to be essential for calcium absorption. Lactase deficiency, however, has a higher incidence in Negroes, and in general osteoporosis is less common in this race than in white people (Trotter *et al.* 1960). Sex hormones still have their advocates. Riggs *et al.* (1969) gave testosterone to osteoporotic men and estrogens to female patients, and reported that the major effect was to reduce bone resorption.

The endocrine hypothesis is an attractive one, but has not yet justified itself. Possibly a low grade of hyperparathyroidism, hardly detectable biochemically, is at work. The results of recent experiments have been interpreted in this way. Pak *et al.* (1969) infused osteoporotic patients with calcium; when the symptoms and calcium balance improved, plasma calcium and phosphate decreased and the bone formation rate (as measured with radiocalcium kinetics) increased. Some of these effects persisted for a month or more after the infusions were stopped. These changes were attributed to increases in formation and decreases in resorption rates in bone and were caused by an increase in calcitonin secretion and a decrease in parathyroid hormone production, due to the hypercalcemia. This interesting hypothesis will no doubt be tested further.

Another interesting possibility is suggested by the work of Harris and Heaney (1969). Working with adult dogs, they found that growth hormone increased the skeletal mass and bone apposition, endogenous fecal calcium loss was decreased, and calcium absorption in the intestine was greatly augmented. Growth hormone stopped endosteal resorption and led to the formation of extensive endosteal bone. They discussed the possible implications of these findings in the treatment of osteoporosis.

As is well known (e.g., Rich and Ivanovich, 1965) reports have indicated that fluoride might have a beneficial effect by improving bone formation in osteoporosis, as fluoride in relatively large amounts is known to cause new bone formation. Recently Henrikson *et al.*

(1970) gave fluoride to dogs with nutritional osteoporosis. No benefits were obtained, the bones were no stronger, and in the mandibular alveolar bone, which showed the most intense osteoporosis, the condition was worsened. (see also Baylink and Berstein, 1967).

It is not yet possible to conclude that one condition only is the cause of osteoporosis. It is obvious that a low calcium intake could cause it, but Hegsted *et al.* (1952) found perfectly healthy people in equilibrium on intakes of 100 and 200 mg per day, so that other factors have to intervene. Almost all workers have found that osteoporotics can absorb and retain calcium perfectly well, but no experiments have lasted long enough to show where they put this calcium. As Garn *et al.* (1967) point out, no matter what the calcium intake, 30 mg of calcium is lost per day after the age of 40. The best preventive is to have a denser bone mass to begin with.

Chapter 12

CALCIUM AND PHOSPHORUS
METABOLISM OF THE TEETH

The teeth consist of three different calcified tissues: enamel, dentin, and cementum. The bulk of the tooth consists of dentin, the crown is covered by enamel, and the roots by cementum.

Enamel

Enamel is the hardest tissue in the body, containing 1.2–4.0% water, 0.2–0.8% organic matter, and 95–97% inorganic matter (Hodge, 1938). Asgar (1956) stated that the enamel of dry teeth contained 36.16% calcium and 16.37% phosphorus. Retief *et al.* (1970) using the method of neutron activation and high-resolution γ-spectroscopy, reported the calcium content of dry enamel to be 31.69%, this method not being applicable to phosphorus.

Enamel is formed by the enamel organ, a complicated structure in which the active cells are the ameloblasts. An organic matrix is laid down first, and is gradually thickened by increments to its final width, becoming calcified at the same time. During this process the organic matrix is withdrawn so that finally there is virtually none in mature enamel, as the above figures show. One practical result of this is that during decalcification in the histological preparation of teeth all the mature enamel is lost.

PROTEINS OF THE MATRIX

The older ideas were that since the enamel organ is ectodermally derived, the protein was a keratin and, as in skin, formed from the cytoplasm of the ameloblast and not secreted. However, it has been shown that the enamel matrix is a true secretion by the ameloblast, since this cell is separated from the matrix by a cell membrane (Watson, 1960; Fearnhead, 1960).

The protein of enamel matrix seems to be unique. Eastoe (1963) reported that fetal enamel protein was quite different from that of adult enamel, collagen, and epidermal and other keratins, and contained no hydroxyproline. Glimcher and his colleagues, in a series of papers, have gone a long way in the elucidation of its structure. The protein has a high proline content and very little if any hydroxyproline (possibly a contaminant); it has a 180° bend in the polypeptide chain at each pyrrolidone residue, and is thus a cross-β-structure (Glimcher et al., 1961). They gave the amino acid composition of the protein of erupted bovine teeth (Glimcher et al., 1964a). During maturation and eruption some enamel proteins are lost, especially those rich in proline and histidine (Glimcher et al., 1964b). Glimcher and Krane (1964) found serine phosphate in the protein of fetal and mature enamel; they thought this might initiate the nucleation of apatite, acting as a bridge linking the structural proteins of the organic matrix to the inorganic crystals. In a further development of this concept, Krane et al. (1965) reported that protein phosphokinase was present in several connective tissues, including the enamel organ. ^{32}P-Labeled serine phosphate was found in a partial hydrolysate of enamel matrix protein after incubation with protein phosphokinase and ^{32}P-Labeled ATP. Seyer and Glimcher (1971) separated four highly purified phosphorus containing polypeptides from the organic matrix of embryonic bovine enamel, containing up to 2.1% phosphorus. Two fractions represented 15–20% of the neutral, pH-soluble proteins. These findings are all in accordance with Glimcher's thesis that nucleation involved phosphorus first.

CALCIFICATION PATTERN

Weinmann *et al.* (1941) considered that the enamel matrix was secreted with about one quarter of its final mineral content and that it awaited a secondary process to transform it into mature tissue. This was based largely on the monograph of Diamond and Weinmann (1940) in which on histological grounds they assumed enamel to be mineralized by a primary followed by a secondary process, the secondary event occurring when the enamel became acid-soluble. Shortly after this, Deakins (1942) and Deakins and Burt (1944), in elegant experiments, in which the results were expressed on a volume basis, showed that there was a gradual linear increase in calcium, phosphorus, and carbonate as the enamel matured, a fivefold increase in inorganic constituents occurring from the softest to the hardest enamel. Rosser *et al.* (1967), working with human and rat molars and using scanning electron probe X-ray emission microanalysis, also found the calcium content of developing enamel to increase linearly with distance from the surface. The isocalcium content contours were not transverse to the incremental lines (as had been stated by Diamond and Weinmann) and no sudden increase in calcium content occurred. Cooper (1968) reported similar findings in pig teeth and also stated that the Ca:P ratio of the calcified enamel matrix did not change in any regular way. In a recent paper, Månsson-Angmar (1971), using quantitative microradiography and studying incisors of stillborn infants, has arrived at exactly the same conclusion. The total volume occupied by mineral salts rose smoothly from immature to mature enamel, and the organic material was lost, also in a smooth linear fashion, from immature to mature enamel.

The subsequent increase in enamel mineral, after the initial calcification, is due to crystal growth (Rönnholm, 1962a). The crystals began as very long, thin plates which increased in thickness and width with increasing mineralization. Mature enamel crystals were 500–600 Å in width and 250–300 Å in thickness (Nylen *et al.*, 1963). Enamel crystals are much larger than those in bone or dentin and are very regularly arranged. Starkey (1971) found that ^{45}Ca was taken up by enamel matrix only to the point where the matrix became acid-soluble. The apparent increase in calcification after this was due to a shrinkage of about 8% in the tissue, no change in overall mineral content occurring.

INITIAL PROCESS OF MINERALIZATION

Avery *et al.* (1961) found that this followed and was closely related to matrix formation, and there was a gradient of radiopacity from the dentin–enamel junction peripherally, which followed a similar pathway to incremental matrix formation. The enamel rods calcified before the interrod substance and the latter provided a pathway for diffusion of fluids containing calcium and phosphorus during calcification. There was no posteruptive increase in mineral content. Several workers stated that crystallization occurs on the fibrous proteins of the enamel matrix, crystal growth following the organic fiber axis (Frank, 1961; Rönnholm, 1962b). The latter worker described a three-dimensional stroma that was revealed after decalcification; it had long, broad septa parallel to crystalline rows, and he considered the crystallites to form on the two broad surfaces of these septa. Perdok and Gustafson (1961) noted a striking correspondence between the repeat distances in the enamel protein and the main lattice translations of the apatite crystal structure. Fearnhead (1963), however, has cautioned that any enamel fibers of a size greater than 20 Å could be artifacts caused by histological technique and felt that it was unwise to assume that the preferred orientation of the crystals was dictated by a preferred orientation of organic fibers.

Work done at that time and subsequently has cast doubt on the fibrous nature of the enamel matrix and the possibility of crystal orientation by fibers. Labeled amino acids, calcium, or phosphorus are laid down incrementally in dentin and this line of deposit is retained, deeper and deeper, as long as the tissue lasts. In enamel, although it is true that the initial calcification occurs at the dentin–enamel junction (Engfeldt and Essler-Hammarlund, 1956; Frank and Sognnaes, 1960), there soon is a diffuse gradient of ^{45}Ca deposition in enamel matrix (Kumamoto and Leblond, 1956). Hammerström (1967) found that when he injected radiocalcium and tetracycline simultaneously, although they were laid down together in newly deposited matrix, they very soon parted company, the calcium being taken up all over the enamel; the tetracycline was not taken up in this way and after 4 days most of the fluorescence had gone.

When the fate of organic compounds was investigated, similar findings were reported. Kumamoto and Leblond (1958) gave ^{14}C-labeled glucose to rats and found the label to become broader and less intense and finally to be lost, in contrast to dentin, where the incremental line persisted. Various labeled amino acids have been used. Hwang *et al.* (1962) found the label after giving [³H] histidine became more diffuse through the enamel matrix with time. Young and Greulich (1963), Cotton and Hefferren (1966), Greulich and Slavkin (1965), and Slavkin *et al.* (1968) have all reported the diffuse, sometimes almost uniform labeling of the matrix after the injection of several labeled amino acids, matrix formed before the injection being also labeled. Greulich and Slavkin analyzed the amino acid deposition on the basis of grain counts and found their results to agree on the whole with the reported chemical analyses except for leucine and serine, other labeled precursors being possibly formed. They considered the enamel matrix to be laid down as a thixotropic gel. Irving (1950a) had previously suggested that the enamel matrix might be laid down as a viscid jelly.

As is well known, fibre formation by fixatives is one of the histologists' problems, and the present writer feels that the fibrous nature of the enamel matrix is still open to question, and the mechanism of apatite crystal formation is not solved.

Shapiro *et al.* (1966) found phospholipids in bovine fetal enamel. Neutral lipids could be extracted before demineralization, but acidic phospholipids could be removed only after this process had been applied, a situation similar to that in bone. They suggested that acidic phospholipids played a role in the calcification process. Irving (1973) examined the molar teeth of young rats during the development stage and found that Sudan black staining of enamel matrix followed closely the mineralization pattern described by Suga and Gustafson (1963) in these teeth, again suggesting the implication of lipids in enamel mineralization.

Dentin

This is a much more elastic tissue than enamel. It contains 10.8–15.7% water, 20.3–22.4% organic matter, and 61–73% inorganic matter (Hodge, 1938). Asgar (1956) reported 30.25% calcium and 13.25% phosphorus in the dentin of dried teeth. The mineral has an apatite structure. The odontoblasts lay down the dental matrix in an incremental manner, the first increment being called predentin. This is not mineralized until a definite time period has elapsed, 24 hours in the case of the rat incisor.

The calcification of dentin matrix takes place by the progressive deposition of mineral (Kumamoto and Leblond, 1956; Takuma, 1960a); in addition, a highly mineralized area encircles the dentinal tubules (Takuma, 1960b), this peritubular calcification occurring after mineralization of the dentin matrix as a manifestation of the maturation of dentin (Atkinson and Harcourt, 1962).

COLLAGEN

The chief protein in the matrix is collagen (Hess et al., 1952). Carneiro and Leblond (1959) found in mice teeth, using tritiated glycine, that the label was over the odontoblasts 30 minutes after injection, in the predentin at 4 hours, and in the dentin matrix at 35 hours and later. The matrix was made in the cytoplasm of the cells, and they did not agree that the cells could trigger collagen formation by inducing extracellular material to precipitate as collagen fibers. It has for long been considered that this was possible in the case of dentin formation, Korff fibers being formed by the subodontoblastic layer and being transformed into collagen on their way to the predentin between the odontoblasts. Recent work by Ten Cate et al. (1970) at the electron microscope level has shown that these fibers, usually visualized with silver, are actually due to impregnation of the ground substance, and that no fibers can be seen. However, in a still more recent paper on initial dentin formation in human teeth at the electron microscope level, Sisca and Provenza (1972) have described collagen fibers which they consider to be Korff fibers. They give a good summary of the controversy about the existence of these fibers, which cannot be considered to be yet settled.

Veis and Schlueter (1964) reported that highly purified dentin collagen contained relatively large amounts of organic phosphorus (16 atoms phosphorus/1000 amino acid residues) at least partially bound to serine as phosphoserine. They considered that the peptide backbone was combined with a side chain (the F component) consisting of oxidized carbohydrate coupled to a phosphoprotein. In a later paper

(Zamoscianyk and Veis, 1966) they characterized the protein as a phosphate-containing sialoprotein and gave details of its composition. Phosphoserine was present in considerable quantities and they thought this phosphate-containing sialoglycoprotein might be involved in the mineralization process. In contrast, corium collagen contained virtually no phosphorus. Earlier it was mentioned that François et al. (1967) had found organic phosphorus in bone collagen, possibly in a similar combination, but the amount present was only slightly above that found in soft tissue collagens.

Although much of the older work showed the presence of glycosaminoglycans in dentin (e.g., Hess and Lee, 1952; Wislocki and Sognnaes, 1950) there is little evidence that they have any direct control of dentin calcification. The only recent suggestion has come from Bevelander and Nakahara (1966), who found granular masses to be extruded by the odontoblasts which they identified as acid glycosaminoglycans, and on which calcification began. It is true that in undecalcified dentin there is a strongly metachromatic line at the dentin–predentin junction, but this can be explained in a number of other ways.

Irving (1963) had shown a sudanophil line at the junction of dentin and predentin, where calcification began, and Shapiro et al. (1966) reported the presence of acid phospholipids in dentin, which could be extracted only after demineralization of the tissue. They hypothesized that the lipids might play a role in dentin calcification. As in all calcifying tissues, sudanophilia is found only where calcification is being initiated, and it is of interest that Savchuck and Burstone (1958) reported the presence of an esterase in areas where dentin was undergoing calcification and from which the sudanophilia was shortly afterwards removed.

Metabolic Activity of the Teeth

Dental structures, after full maturation, are outside almost all vital influences of the body (with the exception of a few processes such as the formation of secondary dentin); having no physiological resorptive mechanism, neither enamel nor dentin can contribute calcium or phosphorus for homeostatic purposes. In addition, fully formed dental tissues are metabolically very inactive. Von Hevesy *et al.* (1937) calculated that the human tooth exchanged about 1% of the dietary phosphorus every 250 days. Von Hevesy and Armstrong (1940) likewise reported that the enamel of the permanent and erupted teeth of cats took up little injected ^{32}P, about one tenth of that of dentin. Volker and Sognnaes (1940) gave ^{32}P to an adult cat by stomach tube; they detected 4.4% of the dose in teeth of which 91% was in the dentin and 2.3% in the enamel. Bone contained four times as much isotope as dentin.

Barnum and Armstrong found the same (1941) and considered that pathways existed for ^{32}P to go from the saliva to the dentin via the enamel, and from the blood to the enamel via the dentin. The main source of ^{32}P to the teeth was from the blood supply to the pulp. They found that the ^{32}P of rat molars was not completely removed by exchange after 116 days. In confirmation of the importance of the blood supply, Gilda *et al.* (1943) reported pulpless teeth to take up much less ^{32}P. Sognnaes and Shaw (1952) have studied the uptake of injected radioactive phosphorus in enamel and dentin of the erupted teeth of monkeys and found that there was a gradient in concentration of ^{32}P, in the case of enamel falling from the exterior to the interior parts and rising from the internal to the external (nearest the pulp) dentin. They attributed these uptakes to salivary ^{32}P in the case of enamel and to the blood radiophosphorus in the case of dentin. Sognnaes *et al.* (1955) reported that the enamel of vital teeth took up more ^{32}P than that of nonvital teeth, so that the pulp appeared to contribute the isotope to enamel.

Much work has been done using the continually erupting incisor tooth of the rat. This, as would be expected from a continually calcifying structure, takes up radioactive calcium and phosphorus with great readiness. Carlsson (1951), using ^{45}Ca, found that the content of the isotope in the incisor rose continually up to 24 days after administration. But this interstitial metabolism is, in the case of dentin, very low compared to that of bone, although the ^{45}Ca returned to the circulation with the resorption of bone gives a persistent activity for up to 10 weeks (Tomlin *et al.*, 1955). Armstrong (1945) found in mature rats that incisal uptake of ^{45}Ca and ^{32}P given together was about equal in enamel and dentin.

Influence of Factors upon Erupting Teeth

In contrast to fully mature teeth, teeth during formation are sensitive to a number of dietary and endocrine factors. Either the continually erupting incisors of rats or mice or molars during the eruptive stage have been usually studied. Calcium, phosphorus, or vitamin D deficiency, or parathyroidectomy, all have similar effects on dentin formation in continuously erupting incisors, and Erdheim in 1906 was the first to report the changes after parathyroidectomy. Histologically, the predentin becomes wider, often with vascular inclusions, and the calcified dentin is irregular and arranged in small calcospherites (interglobular dentin). Becks and Ryder (1931) were among the earliest to report this condition in low phosphorus rickets. The Ca:P ratio of the diet is important in this respect. Gaunt and Irving (1940) found that diets of high Ca:P ratio affected the bones more than the teeth; but if the ratio was low, the reverse occurred, and the dentin ash was reduced. Similar results have more recently been reported by Ferguson and Hartles (1964). When vitamin D is given to rats with low phosphorus rickets, the newly formed predentin is properly calcified, but that existing before the vitamin was given remains unchanged (Irving, 1944), illustrating that dentin has no reparative power.

Several factors causing sudden changes in dentin calcification produce a similar histological picture which has been analyzed by Irving and Weinmann (1948) and called the calciotraumatic response. The last-formed dentin becomes hypercalcified, the existing predentin is not calcified at all, and the next-formed dentin is hypercalcified for a short time. This is sometimes seen in the deciduous teeth of children caused by the adventure of birth, and is called the neonatal line (Rushton, 1933; Schour, 1936a). It is also caused by injections of fluoride (Schour and Smith, 1934) and a number of other agents which can change the calcium and phosphorus environment of the teeth. Applebaum (1943) showed by microradiography that the areas appearing histologically hypo- and hypercalcified were in fact radiolucent and radiopaque. The hypocalcified zone, however, will calcify if the tissue is incubated in a calcifying solution, as has been shown by Eisenmann and Yaeger (1971), so that the effect was not on matrix formation but on the calcifying mechanism.

The effects of changes in the calcium and phosphorus contents of the diet upon the composition of teeth was investigated by Sobel and his group. Sobel and Hanok (1948) reported that, as with bone, the phosphate:carbonate ratios of enamel and dentin were related to those of serum. Using the upper incisor of the rat as their test object, they found that the $PO_4:2 CO_3$ ratio varied under their experimental conditions from 2.08 to 7.72 in enamel, and from 4.40 to 9.31 in dentin, a far higher variation than that seen in bone (1.86–3.33). The Ca:P ratios of the diets were 7.69 or 0.029 and these diets had very low phosphorus or calcium content, respectively. In a subsequent paper Sobel and Hanok (1958) investigated the changes in very young cotton rat incisors and molars. Exactly the same was found, the $PO_4:2 CO_3$ ratios of the blood, enamel, and dentin following each other. The effects were more marked in enamel than dentin in both incisors and molars, and in these experiments the Ca:P ratios of the diets were 10.4 or 0.123.

Experimental Dental Caries

This work had an interesting extension into studies of experimental dental caries in cotton rats. Similar experiments were performed (Sobel *et al.*, 1960) in which animals were put on the same diets that Sobel and Hanok (1948) had used at 16 days of age for 4 weeks. They were then given cariogenic diets with the same calcium and phosphorus content plus vitamin D, for 12–14 weeks. The caries experience was significantly lower in the animals on the high phosphorus diet as compared to the other group. They postulated that high-carbonate teeth were more caries susceptible, since carbonate was preferentially dissolved.

The finding that raising the phosphate of the diet would avert caries in rats is not new and had been reported by Klein and McCollum in 1931. McClure and Miller (1959) found that a number of phosphorus compounds were cariostatic to rats when added to a cariogenic diet. The phosphates had to be soluble and had to be given orally, being almost ineffective by stomach tube. Harris *et al.* (1962) found the cariostatic action of phosphate to be increased if the particles of phosphate were coated with lard, since this caused them to be impacted in the fissures of the teeth. Thus the action of phosphate was certainly a local one in the mouth.

No one has confirmed Sobel's thesis that changes in chemical composition of the teeth were a prerequisite for caries to occur, since caries can easily be obtained with no chemical changes. Wynn *et al.* (1956) and McClure and McCann (1960), using diets with varying Ca:P ratios, could not confirm that any correlation existed between caries experience and tooth analysis. Wynn and his group found that there was less caries when the Ca:P ratio of the diet was lowered, but no change in tooth composition. It is probable that the changes in tooth composition noted by Sobel and his colleagues, while undoubtedly true, were coincidental, and that they were observing the now often confirmed fact that a diet high in phosphate has a cariostatic effect in rats. The diets he used had such extreme Ca:P ratios and contents, that, in addition, tooth composition was changed.

Clinical studies, in which human subjects have been given extra phosphate in the diet, have given conflicting results as far as caries experience is concerned. Some (e.g., Stralfors, 1964; Finn and Jamison, 1967) have reported significant inhibition of caries, but others have had only negative results (Averill and Bibby, 1964; Ship and Michelsen, 1964). This is, however, a field that might be worth pursuing further.

Vitamins

Several vitamins besides vitamin D have characteristic protective effects upon the tooth, but these probably affect matrix formation rather than calcification. In vitamin A deficiency dentin formation is upset, odontoblasts do not regress as they should, and excessive dentin is formed on the labial side of the incisor tooth (Wolbach and Howe, 1925; Schour *et al.*, 1941). Enamel formation is also deranged (Irving and Richards, 1939). The vitamins of the B group do not appear to influence tooth formation. In scurvy a characteristic change occurs, the formation of dentin ceasing and the last part formed being sealed off from the pulp by a hypercalcified zone (Fish and Harris, 1934). The odontoblasts lose their ability to make a calcifiable matrix and change to a structure like the *gerüstmark* of bone (Irving and Boyle, 1952). Both vitamins A and C thus affect tooth calcification as well as that of bone, and in a similar way. Lysine or tryptophan deficiency causes a change in the dentin very similar to that seen in calcium or phosphorus lack (Bavetta *et al.*, 1954).

Endocrine Glands

Some of the endocrine glands besides the parathyroids affect tooth formation, causing changes in calcification, matrix formation, or the growth sequences. Hypophysectomy produces a great retardation in the eruption rate, and as a result the rat's incisor has a folded appearance at the formative end (Becks *et al.*, 1946), but dentin apposition continues so that the pulp cavity is almost obliterated (Schour and van Dyke, 1932). The calcification of the tooth is not changed. Thyroidectomy retards the calcification of dentin (Ziskin and Applebaum, 1940) which becomes virtually uncalcified matrix. Adrenalectomy and gonadectomy interfere with dentin calcification (Schour and Rogoff, 1936; Schour, 1936b) but estrogen administration has no effect on rat or mice teeth, which is of interest when its effects on bone are recalled.

One can conclude that while the fully formed and erupted tooth is unaffected by influences exerted within the body, the forming tooth is very sensitive to changes in calcium and phosphorus metabolism and is under the control of several vitamins and most endocrine glands. It has been found that the dentin of rachitic rats responds exponentially to vitamin D dosage in the same way as does the rachitic epiphysis (Irving, 1944), and also that the dental changes after vitamin D dosage could be detected after 24 hours, 4 days before any change could be seen in the bones. The forming teeth have been largely neglected by physiologists, which is to be regretted since they react so quickly and specifically to many diverse influences.

Chapter 13

EXCRETION OF CALCIUM AND PHOSPHORUS IN THE URINE

Calcium

The daily amount of calcium excreted is very variable, as might be expected, since it is under the control of a number of parameters. Nicolaysen _et al._ (1953), reporting figures in a long-term study of 100 men and women, found on an average that the calcium excreted was from 20 to 25% of the intake, but that while the excretion level might be fairly constant for one individual, it varied considerably from person to person; even in the same individual periods of change could occur for no apparent reason. In more recent work, Harrison and McNeill (1966) studied 6 normal male and female subjects. The urinary calcium varied between 75 and 277 mg/day and seemed to correlate to some extent with the dietary intake (175–2100 mg/day). On the other hand, Parsons _et al._ (1968) found with normal female subjects that the urinary calcium excretion had no relation to the intake. Sutton _et al._ (1971) observed both children and adults and reported very variable figures: in children aged 4–14 years, 14–205 mg/day; and in 8 adults aged 35–63, 128–640 mg/day. The renal clearances also varied just as widely.

As with other ions, calcium is filtered through the glomerular membrane and reabsorbed in the tubules. No evidence has been obtained for calcium secretion by the tubules (Wesson and Lauler, 1959). Chen and Neuman (1955) and Poulos (1957) have reported that more than 99% of the filtered calcium is reabsorbed, the calcium percentage in the glomerular filtrate being almost the same as that in an ultrafiltrate of serum. Unlike phosphorus, calcium is always present in the urine even when the intake is minimal. Older workers thought there was a low or possibly no threshold for calcium excretion (e.g., Wolf and Ball, 1949).

REABSORPTION

The information of the site of calcium reabsorption is quite conflicting. Both Howard et al. (1959) and Wesson and Lauler (1959), using the stop-flow technique, concluded that calcium was reabsorbed in a distal area of the nephron and the latter workers found no evidence for additional absorptive sites. On the other hand, Lassiter et al. (1963), using a micropuncture method, reported that there was reabsorption all along the nephron, but the bulk of the reabsorption took place in the proximal convoluted tubule. Duarte and Watson (1967) loaded dogs with mannitol or saline and also found active calcium resorption in the proximal tubule. It seems at present to be impossible to reconcile these conflicting reports.

A considerable amount of evidence exists which suggests that calcium, sodium, and magnesium reabsorption occur in the same site. Wesson and Lauler (1959) used, as stated above, the stop-flow technique and found areas of calcium and magnesium reabsorption approximately coincident with those for sodium and potassium reabsorption. Walser (1961a) concluded that in diuresis, the free calcium ion clearance was the same as that for the sodium ion, sodium and calcium ions being reabsorbed in the same proportions as in plasma. The tubule cell tended to maintain a constant ratio of sodium to free calcium ions in the tubular fluid, so that there might possibly be competitive binding of calcium and sodium ions at cell membranes. The same concept was advanced by Kleeman et al. (1964), Walser (1961b) concluded that in the absence of hypercalcemia, sodium ion excretion determined free calcium ion excretion. Lassiter et al. (1963), Better et al. (1966), Demartini et al. (1967), Duarte and Watson (1967), and Blythe et al. (1968) all produced evidence supporting this thesis, either for calcium and sodium, or for both these ions and also for magnesium. Demartini and his group suggested that both mono- and divalent cations were similarly handled by the renal tubule. Rahill and Walser (1965) also suggested that beryllium, barium, and radium ions might be reabsorbed by a common transport mechanism with calcium.

Antoniori et al. (1969) thought that calcium and sodium had a common transport system in the proximal tubule and loop of Henle, but different mechanisms in the distal tubule. Massry et al. (1970) produced data suggesting that magnesium, calcium, and sodium competed for a common resorptive site or mechanism in the nephron, but that calcium and magnesium reabsorption were more closely related than that of sodium and magnesium.

However, when the kidney is subjected to stress, the relationship between calcium and sodium reabsorption becomes less clear-cut. Massry et al. (1968a) found that after administration of deoxycorticosterone, the calcium and magnesium reabsorptive mechanisms were still the same, but that for sodium was different. Suki et al. (1968) concluded that calcium and sodium reabsorption was suppressed by chronic administration of mineralocorticoids in the more proximal parts of the nephron, but that sodium reabsorption was enhanced in the distal tubule. Massry et al. (1968b) further reported that parathyroidectomy caused a calcium clearance 4–6 times greater than that for sodium and the interdependence of sodium and calcium clearances was altered. However, calcium infusions caused a competitive inhibition of sodium transport, which might be expected to occur. Hoffman et al. (1969), working with humans, found that giving carbohydrate to fasted subjects caused an increased calcium excretion, but also an increased sodium reabsorption. They considered a different site or mechanism to be involved in sodium excretion compared to that of calcium. Antoniori et al. (1971) reported that massive volume expansion with saline caused a greater increase in calcium and magnesium clearance than in that of sodium. They concluded that during this condition there was a dissociation between the transport of sodium and that of calcium and magnesium. Finally, Brinkman et al. (1971) said that low calcium diets caused the tubule to reabsorb calcium in preference to sodium.

If one were to assume, as Cushny (1917) did many years ago, that the reabsorbed fluid was of constant composition, then these findings would invalidate the concept that calcium and sodium are reabsorbed by a common mechanism. It seems to the present writer that although a common mechanism almost certainly exists, it is capable of adjustment, probably by competitive inhibition, to situations where the relative amounts of these ions may undergo more than usual changes.

Bernstein *et al.* (1963) found in humans, using the ratio of calcium to creatinine clearance as an index, that vitamin D has no effect on calcium clearance.

Williamson and Freeman (1957) stated that acidosis in dogs produced an increased renal calcium excretion, because of an increase in filtered calcium, the reabsorption rate being unchanged. Spencer *et al.* (1966) reported a large calcium loss in starving humans, which they attributed to acidosis and loss of organic acids.

Phosphorus

Phosphorus is filtered through the glomerular membrane and partially reabsorbed in the tubules. When intestinal absorption of phosphorus is reduced, the urinary excretion of phosphorus can fall to very low levels and the reabsorption may be as high as 99%. Longson *et al.* (1956) found that humans fell into two groups as regards handling of phosphorus by the kidney. One group gave results in accordance with the classic T_m hypothesis. In the other group, the phosphorus output was not related to the plasma phosphorus level, and the inulin clearance varied over a wide range. This indicated that the reabsorption of phosphorus increased with the glomerular filtration rate even at high plasma phosphorus concentrations, and they could explain this only by assuming that at any one time a proportion of nephrons must be inactive. As mentioned above, it is possible that not all plasma phosphorus is ultrafiltrable, and Bachra and Wöstmann (1955) considered that more than half of the plasma phosphorus was in the form of complexes which delayed or prevented filtration, and thus the normal clearance values in the literature would be too small to represent ionic phosphorus. As a result of this conclusion, they thought that the amount of tubular reabsorption of ionic phosphorus might not be as high as generally believed. Thompson and Hiatt (1957) found, after infusing phosphate solutions into humans, that there was a pronounced reduction in T_m phosphorus, the degree of tubular reabsorption of phosphorus being correlated with the plasma level of inorganic phosphorus and not with that of calcium.

The site of phosphorus reabsorption has been investigated. Craig (1959) loaded rats with phosphate and got calcium deposits and necrosis in various parts of the tubule. The first part of the convoluted tubule and the collecting tubules were unaffected, but the terminal part of the proximal convoluted tubule and the ascending loop of Henle were severely damaged. On the basis of these results, he suggested that the ascending loop of Henle was the main site of phosphorus reabsorption. Puschett and Goldberg (1969) considered that the monovalent ion $H_2PO_4^-$ was the preferentially transported phosphate species and that the rate of reabsorption was directly influenced by the proximal tubule pH (being lessened by a rise in pH) or by the proximal tubule load of bicarbonate (being decreased when the load of bicarbonate rose) or by both.

POSSIBLE SECRETION OF PHOSPHATE

The question of the site of inorganic phosphate reabsorption brings up the further question as to whether inorganic phosphate is secreted as well as reabsorbed by the tubules. Levinsky and Davidson (1957) took advantage of the renal portal system in chicks to separate tubular from systemic and glomerular activity, and considered that the tubules secreted phosphorus, an effect which was augmented by a direct action of parathyroid hormone upon the tubules. Unfortunately these tubules can also reabsorb phosphorus, so that the results were inconclusive.

Turning to mammals, Barclay *et al.* (1947) claimed to have found phosphorus secretion in dogs, and Carrasquer and Brodsky (1961) thought that secretion on the $H_2PO_4^-$ ion occurred as a mechanism of urine acidification, although Handler (1962) pointed out that their results could be equally explained by reduced tubular reabsorption. Another approach was that of Nicholson and Shepherd (1959), who damaged parts of the renal tubule by chemical means, and concluded that phosphorus was reabsorbed in the first third of the proximal tubule and actively secreted in the distal tubule. Nicolson (1959) reported that distal tubular damage prevented the increased phosphorus excretion seen after injections of parathyroid hormone and considered that parathyroid hormone acted on the distal tubule to stimulate active secretion of phosphorus.

None of the published work since that time has supported the thesis of phosphorus secretion by mammalian tubules. Bronner and Thompson (1961) found the excretory pattern of phosphorus and magnesium to be very similar to that of creatinine, and they considered that a very small proportion of these ions were derived from transtubular flux. Handler (1962) used a variety of methods (loading with sodium phosphate, administration of parathyroid extract, infusions of glucose or *p*-aminohippurate) and was unable to detect any evidence for phosphorus secretion by the tubule. Samiy *et al.* (1960), using the stop-flow technique, stated that parathyroid hormone probably diminished the reabsorption of phosphorus in both the proximal and distal tubules.

Harrison and Harrison (1942) claimed that vitamin D caused an increase in tubular reabsorption of phosphorus. However, Crawford *et al.* (1955) found that in parathyroidectomized animals an opposite effect was obtained and proposed that vitamin D acted by suppressing parathyroid action. Kodicek *et al.* (1961) found, after giving ^{14}C-labeled vitamin D_2, that the vitamin was present in the epithelial cells of the upper two thirds of the proximal convoluted tubule and nowhere else, which they thought might coincide with one site of phosphorus reabsorption. However the data reported elsewhere, suggesting that the kidney is the site of the formation of 1,25-dihydroxyergocalciferol, may well be in line with the observation. The label may not be vitamin D_2, but the dihydroxy derivative.

Gerschberg (1962) found that glucose infusions, which caused glycosuria in humans, reduced tubular phosphorus reabsorption by 20%, and postulated that this fraction of phosphorus shared a common reabsorption site with glucose. Parathyroid hormone had no effect on phosphorus excretion when glucose was simultaneously infused; therefore it seemed possible that this mechanism of phosphorus reabsorption was under parathyroid control.

In this connection, Ferguson and Wolbach (1967) and Wolbach (1970) found in chicks and dogs that phloridzin decreased phosphorus excretion either by blocking secretion or enhancing reabsorption. In the spiny dogfish a great deal of excreted phosphorus is secreted and phloridzin had no effect on this animal's phosphorus secretion. If one can transpose results from one species to another, the effect of phloridzin is on reabsorption. This may, as Ferguson and Wolbach pointed out, be related to the effect of phloridzin in inhibiting glucose reabsorption. The effect of growth hormone may be similarly explained. Abramow and Corvilain (1967) reported that this factor increased phosphorus reabsorption but tended to increase glucose excretion.

Drummond and Michael (1964) found that certain amino acids inhibited tubular phosphorus reabsorption, possibly due to a common reabsorptive site.

Isaacson (1962) produced a novel hypothesis, namely, that phosphorus reabsorption was a purely passive process. He worked with dogs and cooled the body. The Q_{10} of sodium reabsorption was 1.67, but that of phosphorus only 1.08. On applying the Arrhenius equation, the mean apparent activation energy for reabsorption of filtered phosphorus was found to be 1200 cal/mole/degree. This figure is well below the upper limit usually considered to apply to purely passive processes (5000 cal/mole/degree). This concept has not been pursued by other workers.

Magnesium, Calcium, and Phosphorus

As has been pointed out elsewhere, there is evidence that calcium and magnesium are similarly handled by the kidney. In addition, it has been suggested that there is some metabolic relationship between these elements and phosphorus.

Maynard et al. (1958) found that lowering the magnesium of the diet caused a number of deficiency effects, including poor growth, raised serum phosphorus, and calculus formation in the kidney. If the calcium and phosphorus of the diet were simultaneously lowered, these pathological changes did not occur. Other workers have shown that the symptoms of magnesium deficiency are accentuated by raising the dietary calcium or phosphorus or both (O'Dell et al., 1960; Forbes, 1963) and that if the calcium or phosphorus in the diet are raised, the magnesium requirement goes up at the same time (O'Dell et al., 1960; McAleese and Forbes, 1961; Morris and O'Dell, 1963). The deleterious effects of excessive magnesium in the diet could be alleviated by increasing the dietary calcium (Morris and O'Dell, 1963). Both Gitelman et al. (1968) and Meyer and Forbes (1968) reported that the blood and kidney changes caused by magnesium deficiency did not occur after parathyroidectomy. This observation is of interest since it has been suggested that magnesium metabolism may be controlled by the parathyroid gland (MacIntyre *et al.*, 1963). However, if there is a homeostatic mechanism for magnesium, it would seem to be less effective than that for calcium.

Neuman and Mulryan (1971) have found that magnesium is not incorporated into the apatite crystal lattice, but is a surface-limited ion.

——————— *Chapter 14*

KINETIC AND CYBERNETIC ANALYSIS OF CALCIUM METABOLISM

FELIX BRONNER*

Introduction

Traditionally, biologists have approached the problem of function in a reductionist and analytical fashion (Yates, 1971). They have sought explanations and developed descriptions in subcellular and macromolecular terms and have rarely attempted conceptual synthesis beyond qualitative assertions. It is not surprising, therefore, that much of the intellectual excitement in the field of calcium physiology has come from better understanding of the cellular role of calcium (cf. Chapter 15). Nevertheless, attempts, have been made in recent years to describe the fate and biological behavior of calcium from the point of view of systems analysis. Both theoretical and applied descriptions have been published, stimulated by the desire to utilize radioactive tracers which permit the measurement of one-way processes (for a review and listing, see Marshall, 1969). If progress here has been slower than in the analytical aspects, this is partly because few workers can readily manipulate the necessary mathematical tools to provide coherent linear descriptions, let alone nonlinear analyses. Moreover, although there exist some general computer programs with the aid of

*Present address: Department of Oral Biology, University of Connecticut Health Center, Farmington, Connecticut.

which it is possible to generate systematic analyses of whole organism data (e.g., Berman *et al.*, 1962), investigators who might be in a position to accumulate such data often seem to feel uncomfortable about unfamiliar approaches and to prefer more naive interpretations. It is the purpose of this chapter to provide the reader with a brief and simplified description of calcium kinetics and its application to some problems of calcium homeostasis. Perhaps this will help to attract workers into the field who can add the necessary sophistication and develop descriptions appropriate not only to the steady state but also to the transient behavior of the system.

Kinetic Analysis

USE OF TRACERS

A tracer can be defined as a material that has a characteristic which distinguishes it from all other similar materials but which does not affect the system properties under investigation. Radioactive or stable isotopic tracers are now the most widely used. In the case of calcium, the pure β-emitter, ^{45}Ca, with a half-life of 163.5 days, or the γ- and β-emitter, ^{47}Ca, with a half-life of 4.7 days, are the most frequently used tracers. One essential requirement for the use of a tracer is that addition to a system adds negligibly to the mass of the system and does not otherwise disturb it. A second requirement is that the tracer become distributed homogeneously or uniformly in the system at a rate that is rapid in relation to the processes under investigation. For example, if in the system depicted in Fig. 1 the tracer is not distributed uniformly, the drop in tracer amount or concentration will not reflect the process under investigation, i.e., the rate of flow.

It is in fact possible to describe the distribution of the tracer in M in Fig. 1 without stopping flow and to assume only that tracer is distributed homogeneously in the sample being measured, without assuming that any sample of M would give the same measurement. What that then implies is that M is no longer a single, homogeneous compartment, but is made up of a series of such compartments. Figure 2 represents such a possibility. If M is no longer a single compartment, the number of possible models becomes very large. For example, if M is made up of two compartments, there can be 16 possible models, as there may be four modes of entry and exit (Sharney *et al.*, 1965). While theoretically

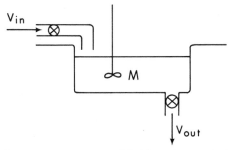

Fig. 1. A simple one-compartment model. M remains constant if $v_{in} = v_{out}$. The stirring device assures homogeneity of M.

If flow is stopped and a tracer (e.g., a dye, D) is introduced into M with stirring and flow resumed after D is uniformly distributed so there is no change in M, measurement of $[D]$ will yield M and the following equations apply:

$$[D]_0 = \frac{D_0}{M} \tag{1}$$

$$[D]_t = [D]_0 e^{-(v_{out}/M)t} \tag{2}$$

Equation (2) can also be written as:

$$2.3 \log_{10} \left([D]_t - \frac{D_0}{M}\right) = -(v_{out}/M)t \tag{3}$$

where

$$[D]_0 = \text{initial concentration of } D.$$
$$[D]_t = \text{concentration of } D \text{ at any time, } t$$

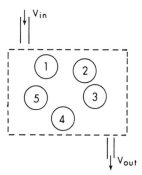

Fig. 2. An extension of the model depicted in Fig. 1. Here M is broken up into a series of compartments. Five compartments are shown but the number can be n. The equations that would apply depend on how the compartments are connected and the direction of flow in relation to them and whether only one or several compartments are accessible to sampling.

one could sample one or several compartments and compare the actual with a host of theoretical time functions and select the most nearly appropriate description as the most likely model, this can become a very tedious and time-consuming exercise, even with high-speed computers. Moreover, it is unlikely that most measurements are sufficiently precise to permit making a reliable distinction between several closely related models. For this reason a model is frequently chosen on the basis of physiological and other considerations and it is a particular model that then is tested. Inevitably different investigators will select different models and controversy in the literature has often centered on certain features rather than on heuristic use of the models. As will be shown, in the case of calcium models, interest has generally centered on the rates of exit and entry or their components, rather than on the detailed interlocking of the compartments and the fluxes between them. However, the magnitude of these rates of entry and exit, particularly of the rate of skeletal calcium deposition, is an intimate function of the model used and can easily vary by a factor of 2. This situation has been used to discredit the systems approach. Yet even the most elegant experiments dealing with the effect of calcium on the conformation and function of a physiologically important protein cannot be used to predict calcium requirements, whereas an estimate of the rate of skeletal calcium deposition may yield such information.

BLOOD SERUM SPECIFIC ACTIVITY

When radioactive calcium is injected into the veins of a mammal, the serum (or plasma) specific activity will decrease as a function of time. The nature of this function has been the subject of much controversy. Two general approaches have been proposed to analyze this time-dependent function: (a) to consider this function a sum of exponentials, and (b) to consider the function a power function.

Let it be said at the outset that neither the exponential nor the power function describes experimental observations adequately over a very long time span. In an exponential function a single term of the multiterm expression becomes dominant with time. Operationally this means that the system then behaves as one undergoing clearance. No long-term data of the behavior of calcium or other bone-seeking nuclides (strontium, barium, radium, etc.) indicate this to be true in the strict sense. Rather the serum-specific activity function gently curves with time, so that if one were able to continue measurements long enough, complete description would always seem to require an additional exponential term.

The power function is a rather poor description of the early portions of the serum-specific activity curve, but becomes better and better as time goes on.

It is not surprising, therefore, that workers concerned with long-term events have tended to favor a type of power function, while those interested in short-term events have gravitated to exponential descriptions. Marshall (1969) has shown that modification of the power function can fit experimental data between 15 minutes and 40 years (!) in some cases. On the other hand, the meaning of such a function in terms of constituent processes is obscure.

One can approach this problem in still another way (cf. Hart, 1967). At any moment the radioactivity in the compartment into which it was injected—usually the serum—is made up of radioactivity that has not yet left the compartment and all that has already returned to it since the beginning of the experiment. If one can only sample the serum these two types—calcium that has not yet left and calcium that has already returned—cannot be differentiated. Some of the radioactivity that leaves the serum is lost by excretion from the body and some is deposited in the skeleton and other calcific deposits. If one measured the total amount of radioactivity excreted and the total amount in the plasma, then, operationally speaking, all radioactivity not accounted for by either measurement must necessarily be "deposited." The difficulty is that this repartition is a time function and that the relative distributions do not reach a steady state within the usual experimental period. Moreover, if one were to wait a relatively long period, the dynamic processes in bone, though relatively slow, would become sufficiently dominant to perturb the system. It is this interplay that results in the complicated time course of the serum specific activity.

To utilize radiocalcium for kinetic studies it is, therefore, necessary to decide on the purpose of the study, since in practice a number of arbitrary decisions have to be made before experimental observations can be turned into specific information.

Investigators have used kinetic studies either to measure specific parameters of calcium metabolism—bone formation, intestinal ab-

sorption, etc.—or to study systems behavior, e.g., calcium homeostasis. From what has been said above, it should be apparent that the
limitations inherent in the kinetic approach have very different effects,
depending on the ultimate purpose of the study. For example, calcium
uptake by bone is the result of a series of processes, each in turn complicated and not well understood. Marshall (1969) has defined calcium
apposition as the process that leads to an increase in bone volume and
calcium augmentation as the process that increases the density of a
given bone-volume element. The respective processes in the opposite
direction are termed resorption and diminution. Calcium entry into
bone is the result of apposition and augmentation processes, both of
which are presumably subject to cellular and homeostatic control.
Whether such control is exerted directly on the process or is the con-
sequence of a cellularly determined structure is as yet entirely conjectural. As Marshall (1969) discusses at length (see also Chapter 9),
the relative importance of each of these processes, apposition *vs* augmentation, is a function of age and of the physiological status of the
animal under study.

Consequently, a value for "bone calcium entry" as measured by
kinetic analysis is not an invariant parameter, but one that varies with
age, nutritional status, sex, etc. With appropriate experimental technique, this value will be the same in similar populations when measured
under similar conditions. The value is not likely, however, to be the
equivalent of that obtained by the common histological techniques
which can estimate only the net difference between apposition and
diminution (cf. Richelle and Onkelinx, 1969). Moreover, bone calcium
entry, as measured by kinetic analysis, is not the same value if estimated
over different time periods.

Similar caveats apply to all other uses one wants to make of the results of kinetic studies. Indeed, perhaps the most effective use one can
make of parameters from kinetic studies is to compare the effect thereon of a variety of experimental situations likely to alter one or several
of these parameters. If this is done, it may be possible to interpret
changes on the basis of known physiological effects and thereby to gain
deeper understanding of these effects. In what follows an attempt will
be made to give a coherent kinetic description and to explore the uses
to which such a description can be put.

A Two-Compartment Open Model

Period of Analysis

As pointed out above, the specific activity of the blood serum (and of other body compartments) is a time-dependent function. If interest in the analysis is focused on system behavior and regulation, the early portions of the function, here termed R_s (identical to the symbol S used by Marshall, 1969), will be of greatest interest, since they reflect short-term processes. On the other hand, if interest is in the skeletal system, then the relatively slow rates and long time periods that seem to characterize many aspects of skeletal calcium behavior make it imperative to deal with the later portions of this function, preferably extending to weeks, months, or even years. From a practical viewpoint it is difficult to measure R_s for more than a few days. However, these practical difficulties are being overcome by more sensitive measurements and by analysis of the body retention curve which is related to R_s (Marshall, 1969).

The very early portions of R_s, i.e., between 0 and 60 minutes, are also difficult to measure, since the concentration of the tracer drops precipitously. Consequently, it is necessary to obtain many measurements, either by frequent sampling or continuous measurement. The former is difficult in rats and other small mammals. It is annoying in man and larger animals. Continuous sampling, e.g., by a flow-through system, is feasible, provided one knows how much of the total flow is being sampled.

It is generally thought, although without analytical or experimental backup, that mixing and redistribution processes tend to dominate in the first few minutes after intravenous tracer injection. For these reasons, most investigators have tried to strike a compromise and have used a model that tended to ignore—either formally or effectively—the first few minutes after tracer injection, but that would suitably account for the experimentally observed time course of R_s for a few days, presumably to include some of the faster of the class of relatively slow bone events.

Bronner and Lemaire (1969) have shown that the time course of the blood plasma-specific activity (R_s) in women and rats can be quite accurately described by a two-termed exponential equation. This equation applies to a period between 1 and 148 hours in people and 2 to 72 hours in rats following intravenous injection. In cattle, a two-termed equation applies between the periods of 2 hours and 5 days following tracer injection (C. F. Ramberg, personal communication). The question whether the equivalent formulation necessarily means process equivalence will be dealt with below.

The blood plasma-specific activity between t_1 and t_2 following an intravenous injection of tracer calcium can be described by an expression of the type

$$R_s = Ae^{-at} + Be^{-bt} \qquad (1)$$

where

   R_s = specific activity (either μCi/mg Ca or % dose/mg Ca)
   t = time (usually hours or days)
   A, B are constants (units: either μCi/mg Ca or % dose/mg Ca)
   a, b = constants (units: T^{-1})

This equation may be thought to have been generated by a two-compartment system. Theoretically it is possible for a two-termed equation to be generated by a system that has more than two compartments. However, in practice this means that several compartments are lumped into one and that during the period of observation the system behaves as if it had only two compartments.

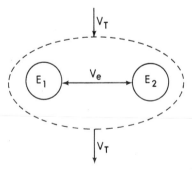

Fig. 3.   A general two-compartment open system. v_e = rate of exchange (units: $M \times T^{-1}$, e.g., mg Ca/day) between compartment E_1 and E_2 (units: M, e.g., mg Ca); v_T = rate of entry or exit into the system (units: mg Ca/day).

Model

The simplest situation is a two-compartment system in steady state with the environment, i.e., where the pool (the sum of the two compartments) neither gains nor loses calcium (Fig. 3). In such a situation, the pool represents the mass (or volume) of calcium into which the tracer would have distributed itself if $v_T = 0$ while the specific activity of E_1 and E_2 became equalized and if tracer had been injected into one compartment only. In practice, pool size is calculated from the differential equations describing the system, since v_T is never zero and since the concentration of the injected tracer is the resultant of redistribution within and loss from the system.

In a crude way one may imagine all of the pool calcium to be divided into two classes, one of which comprises all calcium that turns over with a half-time equivalent to that of the first term of Eq. (1) and the other with a turnover time equivalent to that of the second term of Eq. (1). We shall term these the "more rapidly exchangeable" and "more slowly exchangeable" compartments. It is not easy further to identify these two classes in physiologically meaningful terms. Since the amount of extraskeletal calcium in mammals is smaller than the size of the first compartment, it is clear that the pool calcium comprises calcium of skeletal origin.

Calcium enters the pool by two principal routes: by absorption from the intestine and by resorption from those portions of the skeleton that are outside of the pool. Calcium leaves the pool by three principal routes: by excretion into the urine and in the form of the fecal endogenous calcium, and by deposition into the skeleton. Expressed symbolically:

$$v_T = v_a + v_{o-} = v_u + v_{ndo} + v_{o+} \tag{2}$$

where

v_T = rate of entry into or exit from pool (units: $M \times T^{-1}$, e.g., mg Ca/day)
v_a = rate of calcium absorbed from gut
v_o^- = rate of calcium resorbed from skeleton
v_u = rate of calcium excreted in urine
v_{ndo} = rate of calcium excreted in the stool in the form of fecal endogenous calcium
v_{o+} = rate of calcium deposition in skeleton

The above formulation neglects losses via the skin and via other routes (e.g., milk, semen, menstrual fluid, etc.). These losses are generally agreed to be small in most situations. In any case, terms denoting such losses, if they are measured, are readily incorporated in Eq. (2) (Bronner, 1964).

It is instinctively obvious that if radioactivity is injected into the bloodstream, the rate at which the blood-specific radioactivity decreases is a function of both v_T and v_e, i.e., of the rate of loss from the system (v_T) and of the rate of redistribution within the pool (v_e). In other words,

$$R_s = f(v_T, v_e) \tag{3}$$

It should also be obvious that the actual model chosen to represent the system will determine the numerical solutions. Of the many theoretical two-compartment models that can be constructed, only three

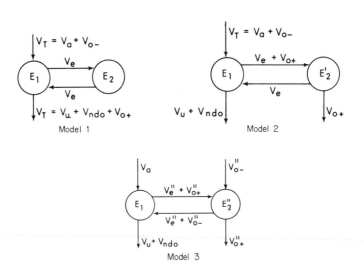

Fig. 4.   Three possible two-compartment open models of calcium metabolism.

will be considered (see Fig. 4). They differ in the way skeletal calcium deposition and resorption are thought to take place in relationship to the two compartments making up the pool.

In Model 1, all undirectional entries and losses (equivalent to v_T) are considered to take place via E_1, the compartment with relatively rapidly exchangeable calcium. In Model 2, all of the calcium destined for skeletal deposition (v_{o+}) flows through and enters the skeleton from the second compartment (E_2'), which contains the more slowly exchangeable calcium. In Model 3, calcium that is resorbed (v_{o-}) also enters the exchangeable pool via the more slowly exchanging compartment (E_2'').

Models 1 and 2 represent two extremes as far as v_{o+} is concerned and Models 1 and 3 represent such extremes with regard to both v_{o+} and v_{o-} (a fourth model, where only v_{o-} but not v_{o+} enters the second compartment, is theoretically possible).

Choice of a given model depends on which fits data best or which is thought to correspond most closely to physiological reality. As can be shown (available on request from the author) Models 1 and 2 yield different values for the second compartment, but identical values for v_e, v_T and the component rates. Model 3 yields higher values for v_T, v_{o+} and v_{o-} and the second compartment, and lower values for v_e. In other words, in Model 3 the relative proportion of the exchangeable and undirectional skeletal processes is altered. Model 3 therefore tends to overcome the "negative resorption problem" (Bronner, 1967; see also Marshall, 1969) and corresponds somewhat more closely to the ideas of long-term "exchange." All of these problems result from the skeleton not constituting a true calcium sink, as does the environment, but one from which calcium returns to the pool with time. It is, therefore, related to the question of experimental period. If the period of observation is long in relation to the lifetime of the organism under study, it is probably a poor assumption to consider the period of observation to represent a steady state. If, however, the period of observation is very short, the derived parameters may not be typical or representative.

Resolution

A numerical example giving detailed resolutions of the three models shown in Fig. 4 is available from the author. The fundamental principle involves resolution of differential equations describing time course of specific activity in the two compartments following tracer injection into first compartment. These are resolved numerically with aid of plasma-specific activity curve considered to be expression of the system. With availability of computers it is relatively simple to develop programs for deriving the best-fitting system equation [Eq. (1)] from experimental plasma data. This should be done for every patient or animal studied. It is not desirable to obtain a best-fitting equation for the population of points as a time function, since without very sophisticated fitting procedures it is difficult to exclude the "out" point which would tend to distort a mean. However, an out point is readily eliminated from a simple time sequence for a single patient or animal.

The system equation is then utilized to calculate compartment sizes (E_1 and E_2, or E_1 and E_2', or E_1 and E_2'') and the rates of undirectional entry and exit (v_T), as well as the rates of movement between compartments (v_e).

The next step involves calculation of the constituent rates making up v_T. The urinary calcium excretion, v_u, can be measured directly on urine collected for several 24-hour periods. Urinary isotope excretion in that period can also be measured. The fundamental relationship that governs isotope loss from a compartment is the differential equation

$$\dot{R}_s = R/v \tag{4}$$

where

$\dot{R}_s$ = the specific activity (e.g., μCi/g) at any moment
          ($\equiv dR_s/dt$)
R = radioactivity lost (μCi/min)
v = the rate of loss (e.g., g/min)

In the case of urinary excretion, v becomes v_u and R becomes R_u, i.e., the radioactivity excreted via and recovered in the urine. $\dot{R}_s$ is the specific activity of the plasma just before filtration; v_u is averaged for the period of investigation ($\overline{v}_u$), and Eq. (4) can therefore be integrated as follows:

$$\int_{t_1}^{t_2} \dot{R}_s = \frac{R_u]_{t_1}^{t_2}}{\overline{v}_u} \tag{5}$$

Since the cumulative urinary calcium and radiocalcium excretions can be determined experimentally, Eq. (5) provides a means of estimating the definite integral of the serum-specific activity without the necessity of knowing the precise time-dependent function of R_s. In other words, even if $R_s(t)$ were a power or some other function, Eq. (5) is true and can be used to estimate the definite integral.

By estimating the definite integral of the plasma specific activity from Eq. (5) it is possible to estimate the average fecal endogenous calcium output, $\bar{v}_{ndo}$, as follows:

$$\int_{t_1}^{t_2} \dot{R}_s = \frac{R_{ndo}]_{t_1}^{t_2}}{\bar{v}_{ndo}} \tag{6}$$

By substituting from Eq. (5) and rearranging, one can write:

$$\bar{v}_{ndo} = \frac{R_{ndo}]_{t_1}^{t_2}}{R_u]_{t_1}^{t_2}} \bar{v}_u \tag{7}$$

The delay between filtration at the glomerulus and entry into the bladder is negligible in balance experiments. The comparable fecal delay is not negligible, however. From a practical viewpoint it is necessary to give a fecal marker at t_1 and again at t_2 and to measure the fecal radiocalcium output in samples between t_1 and t_2, the time periods between which urine is also collected.

With v_T, v_u and v_{ndo} determined, v_{o+} is calculated by difference from Eq. (2) and v_{o-} is determined from the relationship:

$$\Delta = v_i - (v_u + v_F) = v_{o+} - v_{o-} \tag{8}$$

where

Δ = calcium balance ($M \times T^{-1}$, usually mg Ca/day)
v_i = total calcium ingested
v_F = total fecal calcium output

Equation 8 implies that the skeleton is the only calcium storehouse in the body. This may not be entirely true in severe tissue calcification such as myositis ossificans. Experimentally Δ is measured by the balance technique.

PHYSIOLOGICAL SIGNIFICANCE

As already stated, the principal use of the model and its resolution is a heuristic one, i.e., to analyze the system under a variety of conditions so as to gain better understanding of these conditions and also of the model and its limitations. Nevertheless, it may be useful briefly to review the physiological significance of the parameters of calcium metabolism that characterize the model.

The model incorporates parameters that in physiological terms are immediately understandable, i.e., the rates of calcium ingestion (v_i) and excretion (v_u, v_F). It includes others that seem relatively easy to understand but need careful definition (v_{o+}, v_{o-}, v_{ndo}, v_a) and some that seem obscure (pool, E_1, E_2, v_e).

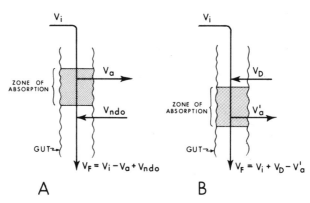

Fig. 5. Two schemes of net calcium movement in the mammalian intestine. In Scheme A, all of the endogenous calcium that enters the intestine is no longer subject to absorption. In Scheme B, all of the endogenous calcium is subject to reabsorption. v_i = amount of calcium ingested ($M \times T^{-1}$, e.g., mg Ca/day); v_F = fecal calcium excreted. If v_i and v_F are identical in both schemes, we can write:

$$\alpha = \frac{v_a}{v_i} = \frac{v_a'}{v_i + v_D}$$

i.e., the fraction of gut calcium absorbed is considered the same. Then:

$$v_{ndo} = v_D - \alpha v_D$$

v_a and v_{ndo}

Figure 5 illustrates two possible models of calcium movement in the gut. In one (Fig. 5A) calcium that enters the bloodstream from the gut by absorption is entirely exogenous, with all calcium leaving the bloodstream for the gut no longer subject to absorption. In the other (Fig. 5B), calcium that enters the bloodstream by absorption is both exogenous and endogenous, all endogenous calcium being subjected to recycling (i.e., reabsorption). These two models represent two extremes. The actual situation in the gut probably is intermediate, as it seems reasonable to suppose that endogenous calcium that enters the gut in the form of succus entericus in the anterior portion of the intestine is more likely to be reabsorbed than endogenous calcium secreted into the posterior portion of the intestine or colon (for further discussion, see Bronner, 1964).

As reëmphasized by Marshall (1969), v_{ndo} (equivalent to his k_F) is directly measurable and represents the net loss of body calcium from the intestine. Physiologically speaking it is the amount of calcium that would enter the gut if there were no recycling. If calcium entered the gut and were reabsorbed as well as food calcium (Fig. 5B), then $v_D[= v_{ndo}/(1 - \alpha)]$ would represent the amount of calcium that would have been secreted into the gut. If endogenous calcium were absorbed more readily than food calcium (but see Schedl et al., 1968, who claim the opposite) then the true v_D would be greater. In a crude way, v_D can be thought of as an estimate of the net flux in the intestine. The validation of this statement requires analysis and measurements beyond the scope of this chapter.

v_a Represents the absorbed exogenous calcium, i.e., that portion of the ingested calcium that is extracted by the gut. The amount of calcium absorbed from the gut in the scheme of Fig. 5B must be greater that v_a in Fig. 5A, since it includes recycled (i.e., reabsorbed) endogenous calcium.

Operationally speaking, the net amount of calcium added to the bloodstream from the intestine is the difference between v_a and v_{ndo}. This difference will be termed S_i and is equivalent to a net absorption rate. Necessarily it must equal the difference between intake and fecal output, i.e.,

$$S_i = v_a - v_{ndo} = v_i - v_F \tag{9}$$

v_{o+} and v_{o-}

Much of the impetus for the use of kinetic analysis has come from the desire to measure calcium deposition in bone. By the same token much of the controversy concerning the kinetic method has come from the difficulty and uncertainty in identifying v_{o+} with histologically defined, intuitively obvious measures of bone calcium deposition. The contributions by Marshall (1969) and Richelle and Onkelinx (1969) are two attempts to deal with this question in depth. Rather than attempt here a detailed discussion, we shall simply emphasize that v_{o+} represents the calcium lost from the pool by routes other than urinary or fecal endogenous excretion. In a nonlactating, normal individual, virtually all of the calcium that leaves the pool by v_{o+} ends up in the skeleton. What fraction is in fact made into bone mineral with substantial sojourn time, what fraction is lost in a matter of a few days or weeks, which is subject to recrystallization and redeposition in the skeleton—all of these important questions are outside of the type of kinetic analysis here proposed, because they demand study of the skeleton proper. The kind of question one can ask is whether v_{o+} and v_{o-} are subject to regulation and how they vary under a variety of conditions. Whereas v_u is the same, whether measured kinetically or by classic balance technique, v_{o+} can only be measured kinetically. Even histological observations, when transformed into estimates of bone formation, become kinetic measures and appropriate comparisons between these two approaches, though important, are difficult and uncertain (Marshall, 1969; Richelle and Onkelinx, 1969). Except for the understandable, but still instinctive preference for a kinetic measure based on direct visual observation, there is little reason to prefer one over the other kinetic estimate. Moreover, from studies with collagen (Lapière et al., 1966) it is becoming increasingly apparent that synthesis and degradation considerably exceed net synthesis. Therefore, the frequently voiced objection that "bone formation" rates calculated from calcium turnover studies are unrealistically high may no longer be entirely valid.

Pool and v_e

As already implied in the preceding discussion, the notions of the calcium pool, its constituent compartments and the rate of flow between them are least readily related to intuitively obvious physiological parameters. For this reason it would be particularly interesting to study the pool under a variety of conditions known to affect calcium metabolism. Very few such studies have been published.

Formally speaking, all body compartments with calcium turnover rates equal to or smaller than the turnover constant of the first compartment, v_e/E_1, will be lumped into the first compartment and all with a turnover constant between v_e/E_1 and v_e/E_2 will be lumped into the second compartment. For example, detailed analysis of the behavior of calcium in skeletal muscle (Gilbert and Fenn, 1957) has shown that muscle calcium is divided into three compartments, one of which appears to have a rather slow turnover constant. On kinetic grounds this third muscle compartment is likely to be part of E_2, yet its size in relation to E_2 is small. This can be demonstrated as follows: In adult man, muscle constitutes about 40% of body weight and has a calcium concentration of about 2.6 mg/kg fresh tissue (Widdowson and Dickerson, 1964). Bronner and Lemaire (1969) found E_2' (i.e., the second compartment analyzed according to Model 2, Fig. 4) to average 1725 mg Ca. The women in question weighed about 60 kg on the average, so that their total muscle Ca was only about 125 mg, of which probably only about one third (Gilbert and Fenn, 1957; Bloomquist and Curtis, 1972) or 40 mg was in the very slow compartment. Clearly this represents a tiny fraction of E_2', so that the identification of E_2' with some skeletal calcium is only slightly inaccurate.

INTERSPECIES COMPARISONS

In Table I are listed the kinetic parameters derived from two-compartment analyses of the plasma calcium disappearance curve of three species. The table is intended to be representative rather than record all available data and reflects differences in sex and age.

Of great interest is the fact that even though these three species differ so widely in life span and size the rate constants k_e, k_T, k_{o+} are so similar. These constants characterize three physiologically important processes, the rate of exchange between the two calcium compartments, the overall turnover of the pool, and the fraction of the pool that goes to bone. Therefore it seems reasonable to conclude that similar processes occur in all three species and that these processes

TABLE I. INTERSPECIES COMPARISON OF KINETIC PARAMETERS OF CALCIUM METABOLISM[a]

Species	Human		Bovine			Rat		
Sex	F[b]	M[c]	F[d]	F[d]	F[d]	M[e]	F[b]	F[b]
Age (years)	56.5	71.1	0.5	1.0	5.0	0.18	0.33	0.83
Wt (kg)	65	70.8	86	353	403	0.23	0.17	0.30
No. studied	6	10	2	3	4	30	14	8
Period of validity (days)	6	8	5	5	5	3	3	3
Pool parameters								
Compartment E_1 (mg)	1640	2050	11,100	23,370	15,750	27	23	11
E_1 (mg/kg BW)	25	29	129	66	40	117	135	37
Compartment E_2 (mg)	1730	2630	71,800	101,900	26,100	136	125	31
E_2 (mg/kg BW)	27	37	836	297	64	591	735	103
Pool, $E_1 + E_2$ (mg)	3370	4680	82,900	125,270	41,850	163	148	42
$E_1 + E_2$ (mg/kg BW)	52	66	965	355	104	708	870	140
Exchange rate, v_e (mg/day)	4270	3250	20,000	28,970	17,550	104	79	42
v_e/kg BW (mg/day $\times$ kg^{-1})	66	46	234	82	44	452	465	140
$v_e/E_1 + E_2$, rate constant, k_e (day^{-1})	1.3	0.7	0.24	0.23	0.42	0.64	0.53	1.0
Unidirectional fluxes								
v_T (mg/day)	722	714	20,700	43,400	16,700	85	71	31
v_T/kg BW	11.1	10.1	242	125	41	370	417	103
Rate constant, k_T (day^{-1})								
$\quad(v_T/E_1 + E_2)$	0.22	0.22	0.25	0.35	0.40	0.63	0.48	0.74
v_{o+} (mg/day)	400	418	19,100	39,600	12,700	78	61	15
v_{o+}/kg BW (mg/day $\times$ kg^{-1})	6.2	5.9	224	114	32	339	359	50
Rate constant, k_{o+} (day^{-1})								
$\quad(v_{o+}/E_1 + E_2)$	0.12	0.09	0.23	0.32	0.30	0.48	0.41	0.36

[a] All analyses are based on Model 2, Fig. 4, except the data of Cohn et al. (1965), which were derived from Model 1, Fig. 4. [b] From Bronner and Lemaire (1969). [c] From Cohn et al. (1965). [d] From C. F. Ramberg, personal communication. [e] From Sammon et al. (1970).

are brought into evidence by the type of kinetic analysis of calcium metabolism described in this chapter.

Although not enough data are listed in the table to permit firm conclusions regarding age, some trends are of interest. For example, if one assumes a human life span of 80 years and a bovine one of 15 years and then plots the ratio of E_1/E_2 as a function of the fractional life span, the data for the women and cows follow an exponential-type curve. This is also true for female rats (assumed life span: 2 years), but their plateau is much lower. Therefore the exchangeable calcium pool appears to shrink with age, particularly in the case of the second compartment (E_2), all of whose calcium is thought to be skeletal. Both on an absolute and fractional basis the skeletal calcium that participates in metabolic processes thus decreases significantly with age. This diminution is more important in humans and cows than in rats. In other words, the rat seems to have a much higher rate of calcium metabolism than the other two species (cf. Bronner and Lemaire, 1969).

Another way to look at this is to plot k_T and k_{o+} as a function of life span. When this is done for women and cows there is a clear suggestion of a peak at about 15–20% of life span (corresponding to about 12–16 years in women and 2.3–3 years in cows) with an exponential drop-off thereafter. The data on rats in Table I are insufficient to show such a peak, but unpublished data on rats (S. I. Chang and F. Bronner) support this possibility.

A comparison of the various parameters on a kilogram body weight (BW) basis (Table I) is also useful, since it shows what has long been suspected, namely, the marked decrease with age of the intensity of calcium metabolism. However, such comparisons are valid only if the calcium content of the body and its compartments are similar in the species being compared. If the logarithm of v_{o+}/kg BW is plotted against age and expressed as a fraction of the life span, the values for the women and cows again fall on a single curve that looks like a set of exponentials with a drop of about two orders of magnitude for the entire life span. When this is done for rats the values are much higher, but the drop-off with age appears greater.

It is apparent, therefore, that this type of analysis can yield useful information and insights and may be of help in providing a quantitative basis for comparative studies. Obviously many more data are needed to permit detailed quantitative information.

Cybernetic Analysis

One of the principal uses to which kinetic analysis can be put is to develop and test models of regulation. For example, one might suppose that intenstinal absorption (v_a) and skeletal deposition (v_{o+}) of calcium are related. A number of such studies have been done and the general conclusion is that v_{o+} is relatively independent of v_a (Bronner and Aubert, 1965; Schwartz *et al.*, 1965; Phang *et al.*, 1969). To test a variety of such relationships it is useful first to have developed some model of regulation and then to see whether experimental observations support the model. In what follows one such model of calcium homeostasis will be analyzed. Whereas a number of kinetic approaches have been proposed, the cybernetic model to be discussed is the only quantitative model of calcium homeostasis that has been proposed so far. It is to be hoped that future work will refine and modify this model. The model moreover is based on steady-state relationships, whereas regulation of plasma calcium *in vivo* is effected by transient processes, of which steady-state relationships are only resultants.

THE MODEL

Three systems are involved in plasma calcium regulation: the gut, the skeleton, and the kidney. If plasma calcium is to remain at or near a given value—typically 2.5 mM in mammals—the sum of inputs and outputs from the three systems must necessarily equal zero. In the growing animal, calcium is added to the plasma by intestinal absorption and extracted from plasma by renal excretion and net deposition in the skeleton. When the skeletal calcium balance is negative, as in aging animals or in certain disease states, the skeleton adds calcium to the blood; but in the normal situation, the skeletal calcium balance varies from positive to near zero. Urinary calcium excretion (v_u) and skeletal calcium balance (Δ) tend to vary directly with calcium absorption. For example, one can vary net calcium absorption (S_i) in growing rats at will simply by raising or lowering the calcium content of an otherwise unchanged diet (Bronner and Aubert, 1965). Consequently, v_u and Δ of these animals will vary similarly and in the same direction as S_i. It is reasonable to classify the gut as a system whose output tends to disturb the plasma calcium and to classify the kidney and skeleton

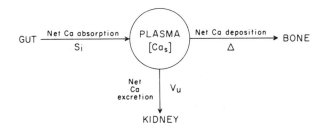

Fig. 6. Regulatory classification of parameters of calcium metabolism. (From Bronner *et al.*, 1970, and reproduced with permission of the publisher.)

as systems whose outputs regulate or control plasma calcium (Aubert and Bronner, 1965). Figure 6 is a schematic representation of this statement.

The net output or signal of a system is the resultant of constituent signals, i.e., $\Delta = v_{o+} - v_{o-}$, $S_i = v_a - v_{ndo}$; $v_u = v_{fi} - v_r + v_s$. One need not necessarily classify constituent signals in the same way as net signals, but for the sake of simplicity constituent signals have been classified in the same manner as the net signals.

Another objection that can be raised to this approach relates to possible feedback paths that may exist between the systems. The literature contains many suggestions of a feedback path between gut and skeleton. However, with the possible exception of the work on the role of 1,25-dihydroxycholciferol (Boyle *et al.*, 1971), none of these reports indicates the existence of an acutely functioning feedback path. For this reason the model to be discussed here will not take such a feedback path into account.

Finally, it should be emphasized that classifying the gut as a disturbing system is not meant to imply that it is not subject to control. All biological systems characteristically contain many highly sophisticated

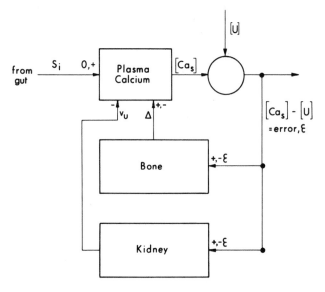

Fig. 7.   Diagram of plasma calcium regulation, with hormonal controls omitted (as in thyroparathyroidectomized animals):

S_i =   net Ca absorption from gut, $M \times T^{-1}$
v_u =   urinary Ca excretion, $M \times T^{-1}$
Δ =   net bone Ca balance, $M \times T^{-1}$
$[Ca_s]$ =   plasma calcium concentration, $M \times V^{-1}$
$[U]$ =   plasma calcium reference value, $M \times V^{-1}$
ϵ =   error ($[Ca_s] - [U]$)

S_i is the disturbing signal, v_u and Δ are the controlling signals with bone and kidney responses proportional to the error, ($[Ca_s] - [U]$)

(From Bronner, 1973, and reproduced by permission of the publisher.)

controls. However, the output of a regulated system can still function as a disturbing signal for another system and this is the intent of the classification used here.

Figure 7 depicts the simplest control diagram relating intestinal calcium absorption, net skeletal calcium deposition, and net kidney calcium excretion to plasma calcium maintenance. The diagram omits hormonal controls and does not show constituent signals. It is drawn according to the convention of linear control systems. When calcium enters the bloodstream via absorption from the intenstine, it tends to raise the plasma calcium concentration $[Ca_s]$, which is drawn as a signal that is being compared in a comparator with a "set" or "reference" value $[U]$. This is the value at which the body is attempting to hold the plasma calcium. The difference between actual plasma calcium and reference value is termed the "error signal."

It is the error signal that actuates the two controlling systems, bone and kidney. When the error is positive, i.e. when the plasma calcium concentration $[Ca_s]$ exceeds the reference value, bone responds by a positive net deposition, i.e., more calcium is being laid down than removed and the mass of bone calcium increases. At the same time, the kidney responds by increased net calcium excretion, i.e., v_u increases. If the error is negative, i.e., when $[Ca_s]$ drops below the reference value $[U]$, bone responds by causing the amount of calcium being resorbed to exceed that being laid down, i.e., the bone balance becomes negative. The kidney responds by diminishing v_u to near zero. It is assumed that in the absence of hormonal controls, as in thyroparathyroidectomized animals, the two controlling systems, bone and kidney, respond in direct proportion to the error, i.e., as proportional controls. This is the simplest situation, but one that still requires experimental proof. Indirect evidence in man (Hall *et al.*, 1969) and the rat (Sammon *et al.*, 1970) on the linear relationship between disturbing and controlling signals adds weight to the supposition that the fundamental control is proportional, but direct proof would require data of a precision not yet available.

The diagram in Fig. 7 contains formulations which are as yet far removed from what is known. For example, nothing is known of the nature of the transducers, i.e., the mechanisms by which mass flows are converted to signals. One could speculate that a rise in the plasma calcium leads to a rise in the calcium filtered at the glomerulus. This rise in turn could cause a conformational change in a specific kidney cell membrane protein, as a result of which calcium reabsorption in the proximal tubule could be diminished. In that case, the specific membrane protein would serve as a transducer. The conformational change would then be the transducer mechanism. In turn that change could cause less calcium flow, either by restricting pore size or by slowing a pumping mechanism. In that case the transducer would be closely coupled to the flow mechanism. Intervention of a chemical messenger would represent somewhat looser coupling.

One could also object to the diagram of Fig. 7 by pointing to the absence of a known comparator. As in the case of the transducer, one can imagine a molecular mechanism, such as a conformational change, that would effectively serve as a comparator. It is not necessary to identify a single organ or mechanism to be able to use a comparator as a symbol in a control diagram. The identification of calcium binding proteins in intestine (Wasserman and Taylor, 1969; Fullmer and Wasserman, 1972) and kidney (Sands and Kessler, 1971) makes it possible now to imagine fairly specific molecular mechanisms that, taken together, could function as a comparator.

The relative importance of kidney and bone in overcoming the disturbing signal varies in different species and is a function of age. For example, in young, growing, male rats, only 2% of the incoming disturbing signal is handled by the kidney (Sammon et al., 1970), whereas in adult women the kidney handles 23% and bone only 67% (Hall et al., 1969). This is illustrated by the following set of equations:

In young growing rats

$$v_u = 0.3 + 0.02 \, S_i \qquad (10)$$

$$\Delta = -0.3 + 0.98 \, S_i \qquad (11)$$

In women

$$v_u = 114 + 0.23 \, S_i \qquad (12)$$

$$\Delta = -114 + 0.77 \, S_i \qquad (13)$$

where

v_u = urinary Ca excretion
Δ = body or skeletal Ca balance
S_i = net intestinal absorption
(units: mg Ca/day)

Equations (10–13) were derived for normal persons and animals, i.e., with all hormonal controls intact. In rats, neither parathyroid ablation (Sammon *et al.*, 1970) nor ablation of the calcitonin-producing cells (Sammon *et al.*, 1969) produced a significant shift in the hierarchical relationship of bone and kidney; in both instances bone handled 95% or more of the incoming disturbing signal. Incomplete, unpublished data (F. Bronner and S. I. Chang) on older rats indicate that with age the kidney in rats, as in humans, assumes greater regulatory significance, but does not assume an importance equal to that in man.

Figures 8 and 9 illustrate the regulatory role of the kidney in a somewhat different way. Here, instead of looking at the increase in either v_u or Δ as a function of S_i, the ratio of v_u/S_i is plotted against S_i. In other words, Figs. 8 and 9 attempt to evaluate the overall importance of urinary calcium excretion over the normal or usual ranges of calcium intake and balance. This approach shows that on an absolute basis the kidney in the rat handles only 2–8% of the net intestinal calcium absorption, whereas in women the kidney handles at least 60% of the net amount absorbed. In the rat, therefore, the skeleton is the major system regulating plasma calcium, whereas in adult humans the kidney is at least as important as the skeleton.

HORMONAL CONTROLS

As pointed out above, removal of endogenous parathyroid hormone or calcitonin has no effect on the relative importance of bone and kidney in the rat. However, as will be shown, the hormones modify the nature of the error control and their action modifies the relationship of the constituent signals. No such data are as yet available for humans.

Parathyroid Hormone

The biochemical and tissue actions of parathyroid hormone have already been discussed (Chapter 11). The discussion that follows deals with the regulatory function of parathyroid hormone.

Parathyroidectomy leads to the well-known drop in plasma calcium level and to a decrease in the intensity of the various parameters of calcium metabolism (Sammon *et al.*, 1970). In a simple man-made control system, where positive and negative errors are handled by the same corrective mechanisms, one might imagine a situation where removal of an agent such as a hormone could lead to a uniform drop in

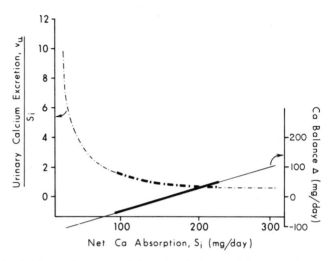

Fig. 8.   Calcium balance, Δ, and the ratio of urinary calcium excretion, v_u, to net calcium absorption, S_i, as a function of net absorption in women. The plot is based on Eqs. (12) and (13) of the text (Hall et al., 1969). The usual range (-50 mg Ca/day $< \Delta < +$ 50) is shown by the heavy lines.

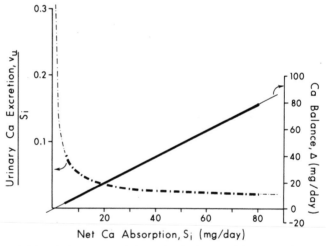

Fig. 9.   Calcium balance, Δ, and the ratio of urinary calcium excretion, v_u, to net calcium absorption, S_i, as a function net absorption in rats. The graph is based on Eqs. (10) and (11) of the text (Sammon et al., 1970). The usual range of values ($+5$ mg Ca/day $< \Delta < +80$) is shown by the heavy lines.

intensity of the parameters of a system. Applied to parathyroid function, this statement would mean that a parathyroidectomized animal would be able to handle a rise or a drop in plasma calcium as well as a normal animal. Intuitively one knows this is not true; rigorous experimental demonstrations have been few.

Equations (14) and (15) provide a quantitative demonstration that plasma calcium regulation is much less precise in the animal without functioning parathyroid glands than in the intact animal:

$$[Ca_s] = 6.02 + 0.021 \, S_i \tag{14}$$

$$[Ca_s] = 10.80 + 0.0021 \, S_i \tag{15}$$

Equation (14) describes plasma calcium (in mg Ca/100 ml) as a function of net calcium absorption (S_i, mg Ca/day) in surgically parathyroidectomized (PTX) animals and Eq. (15) describes this relationship in normal rats.* In the normal rat a calcium load of 100 mg/day from the intestine raises the steady-state plasma calcium to 11 mg/100 ml, or by less than 2%. In the ablated animal a comparable load would raise the steady-state plasma calcium to 8 mg/100 ml, or by 33%. Clearly the PTX animal is less able to regulate his plasma calcium around a steady value. This is also brought out by acute loading studies. When PTX animals received an intraperitioneal calcium load (Bronner et al., 1968) the acute plasma calcium error—i.e., the difference between plasma calcium in the absence of a load and at any moment following administration of the load—was greater than in normal animals. Moreover, it took appreciably longer in the PTX than in the normal animals for the plasma calcium to return to its preload value.

That PTX animals are less able than normal animals to handle a positive error is also brought out by experiments of Copp et al. (1965). These investigators showed that PTX animals on a very low phosphate and moderate calcium diet had greater hypercalcemia than normal animals on this diet.

Quantitative data on the relative ability of normal and parathyroidectomized animals to handle negative errors—as when the plasma calcium is depressed by EDTA infusions—have not been published. Nevertheless, Copp's studies with EDTA infusions of thyroparathyroidectomized dogs (1957, 1960) indicate, as one might expect, that

---

*All equations for normal and PTX animals are taken from Sammon et al. (1970).

ablated animals are less able to handle negative errors than the normal organism.

Thus, parathyroid hormone contributes to more precise plasma calcium regulation and permits overcoming both positive and negative errors of plasma calcium more rapidly.

Nevertheless, the fact that even in ablated animals the plasma calcium returned to the preload value relatively rapidly (Bronner *et al.*, 1968; Sammon *et al.*, 1970) and that the parathyroidectomized animal can maintain a given plasma calcium value in direct relationship to the calcium input [Eq. (14); Copp, 1960] is clear indication of controls capable of functioning in the absence of the parathyroid glands. Consequently, the parathyroids contribute to, but do not exert, sole regulation of plasma calcium. Clearly such regulation must involve error sensing, parathyroid hormone release, and action on the target tissues, bone and kidney. It is these tissues that regulate plasma calcium. How then is bone and kidney regulation of plasma calcium modified by parathyroid hormone?

Since skeletal entry (v_{o+}) and release (v_{o-}) of calcium are the constituent processes of the skeletal calcium balance, Δ [Fig. 6; Eq. (8)], it is reasonable to suppose that their intensity is modified by parathyroid hormone action. Moreover, since parathyroidectomy leads to a lower steady-state plasma calcium level and since plasma calcium regulation is less precise, it is not unreasonable to suppose that the parathyroid hormone acts on the cellular processes leading to v_{o+} and v_{o-} in a way so as to modify their relationship. This is indeed the case. Equations (16–19) describe the relationship between the constituent controlling signals, v_{o+} and v_{o-}, on the one hand, and the disturbing signal (net calcium absorption, S_i), on the other, in both normal and parathyroidectomized rats:

$$v_{o+} = 67.2 + 0.11 \, S_i \tag{16}$$

$$v_{o-} = 67.5 - 0.87 \, S_i \tag{17}$$

$$v_{o+} = 36.5 + 0.29 \, S_i \tag{18}$$

$$v_{o-} = 36.9 - 0.69 \, S_i \tag{19}$$

(units: mg Ca/day)

Equations (16) and (17) apply to normal and Eqs. (18) and (19) to

PTX animals.* In the normal animals, as net absorption increases, v_{o-} goes down much more than v_{o+} goes up. In other words, to maintain its plasma calcium near 10.8, the normal rat, when faced with significant calcium entry from the gut, diminishes mostly bone calcium mobilization, with only a very modest increase in bone calcium deposition. However, when deprived of its parathyroid hormone, the rat faced with a positive calcium load is less able than the normal animal to reduce bone resorption.

On the other hand, when the load is negative, as would be the case when plasma calcium is removed by dialysis or EDTA treatment, the PTX animal would be able to respond less well. This is apparent when Eqs. (17) and (19) are compared. It has also been demonstrated in acute studies (Copp, 1960). Thus parathyroid hormone magnifies the regulatory importance of v_{o-}.

It is interesting to note that the overall regulatory role of the skeleton in the rat is unaffected by parathyroidectomy. This has already been alluded to and can be appreciated by subtracting Eq. (17) from Eq. (16) and Eq. (19) from Eq. (18), as follows:

$$v_{o+} - v_{o-} = 0.3 + 0.98 \, S_i = \Delta \tag{20}$$

$$v_{o+} - v_{o-} = -0.4 + 0.98 \, S_i = \Delta \tag{21}$$

In other words, whether or not parathyroids are present in the growing rat, the primary hierarchical role of the skeleton remains unchanged.

As already stated, parathyroidectomy in the rat has no effect on the proportion of the incoming distributing signal handled by the kidney, nor on the relative importance of kidney and bone. A comparison of Eq. (20) with Eq. (21) shows that parathyroidectomy failed to affect the hierarchical importance of bone. However, from Eqs. (16–19) it is apparent that parathyroidectomy had a considerable effect on the relative regulatory role of v_{o+} and v_{o-}. Therefore, by measuring only v_u as a function of S_i we cannot know what effect parathyroidectomy had on the relative importance of renal calcium filtration and reabsorption. From the data of Kleeman et al. (1961) it is evident that renal calcium reabsorption is increased by parathyroid hormone action, at

*All equations for normal and PTX animals are taken from Sammon et al. (1970).

least in man and the dog. However, no data have been published to permit quantitative evaluation of this effect, as done in Eqs. (16–19).

The effects of parathyroid hormone or plasma calcium regulation may therefore by summarized as follows:

1. Parathyroid hormone is released in proportion to a negative error in the plasma calcium ($[Ca_s] - [U]$).

2. The released hormone acts on bone to cause increased calcium release into the plasma. When bone is under parathyroid hormone dominance, it exerts its control over plasma calcium almost entirely by way of v_{o-}. Both v_{o+} and v_{o-} are much higher in bone under parathyroid dominance than in bone not under this endocrine influence.

3. The hormone also causes an increase in calcium reabsorption in the kidney. Just as the importance of the kidney differs at various ages and in different species, so the regulatory significance of parathyroid modulation of renal calcium reabsorption may vary with age and species.

4. The combined effects of the hormone on bone and kidney regulation of plasma calcium are such as to reduce the steady-state plasma calcium error, $\varepsilon = [Ca_s] - [U]$, to zero.

5. The metabolic effects of the hormone on bone tissue result in more precise control, not only of negative but also of positive errors of the plasma calcium. This applies to both transient and steady-state errors. These statements form the basis of the regulatory diagram shown in Fig. 10. As in Fig. 7, mass flows are converted to signals in each of the organ systems, but the nature of the transducers is not known.

In the model, a negative error is drawn as actuating the parathyroid glands to release hormone that acts on bone and kidney. In addition, as in Fig. 7, both positive and negative errors are shown acting directly on bone and kidney. Bone responds to negative errors by increasing v_{o-} more than v_{o+} and to positive errors by decreasing v_{o-} more than v_{o+}. This differential is accentuated by parathyroid hormone.

Kidney responds to a negative error by decreasing v_u and to a positive error by increasing v_u. The precise relationship between v_r and $v_{fi}(+v_s,$ if v_s exists) and the effect of parathyroid hormone thereon are not known, though v_r is under parathyroid control.

The plus, minus, and zero symbols in the diagram merely indicate direction of flow. For example, v_{o+} is positive with respect to bone and negative with respect to plasma calcium. The signs do not mean that a

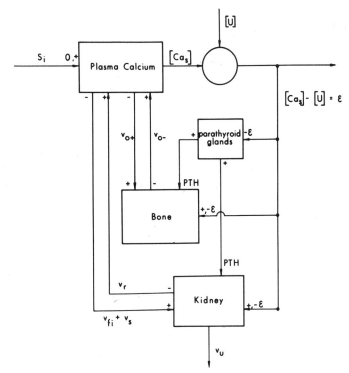

Fig. 10. Diagram of plasma calcium regulation including parathyroid hormone (PTH) action. Other hormonal controls omitted.

$S_i =$ net Ca absorption from gut, $M \times T^{-1}$
$v_{o+} =$ calcium deposition in bone, $M \times T^{-1}$
$v_{o-} =$ calcium resorption or withdrawal from bone, $M \times T^{-1}$
$[Ca_s] =$ plasma calcium concentration, $M \times V^{-1}$
$[U] =$ plasma calcium reference value, $M \times V^{-1}$
$\epsilon =$ error, $([Ca_s] - [U])$
$v_u =$ urinary calcium excretion, $M \times T^{-1}$
$v_{fi} =$ calcium filtered in kidney, $M \times T^{-1}$
$v_s =$ calcium secreted in kidney, $M \times T^{-1}$
$v_r =$ calcium reabsorbed in kidney, $M \times T^{-1}$
PTH = parathyroid hormone

S_i is the disturbing signal, v_{o+}, v_{o-}, v_r, v_{fi}, v_s are the controlling signals, with bone and kidney responses proportional to either the positive or negative error, $\epsilon = ([Ca_s] - [U])$; the net controlling signal of the kidney is $v_u = v_{fi} - v_r + v_s$ (in all likelihood, v_s is zero in mammals); the net controlling signal of bone is $\Delta = v_{o+} - v_{o-}$

(From Bronner, 1973, and reproduced by permission of the publisher.)

positive error signal necessarily evokes a positive flow in the controller. Indeed, as shown by Eqs. (16–19) and stated above, a positive error signal causes more a decrease in v_{o-} than an increase in v_{o+}.

It is important to point out that whereas parathyroid hormone release occurs in proportion to a negative error signal only, the metabolic effects of the hormone on bone and kidney are such as to lead to more precise error control, whether the error is positive or negative.

As a result of the action of parathyroid hormone, steady-state error of plasma calcium is virtually absent [cf. Eq. (15)] and acute error correction is significantly improved (Bronner et al., 1968). In man-made linear control systems, the addition of an integral to a proportional control eliminates steady-state error and minimizes the error-time curve without leading to overshoot (Goldman, 1960). Consequently, it seems reasonable to propose that parathyroid hormone adds an integral control to the proportional control due to bone and kidney, when the latter are not under parathyroid dominance (Aubert and Bronner, 1965).

The preceding statement does not contradict the now well-established proportional relationship between plasma calcium and parathyroid hormone level (Sherwood et al., 1968). Hormone release may well be proportional; the effect of the hormone can still be to provide an added integral control over plasma calcium.

Since parathyroid hormone probably has little or no effect on calcium absorption (Chapter 11), it was unnecessary to deal with the effect of the hormone on the intestine. The hormone has, however, a significant positive effect on urinary phosphate excretion, probably by diminishing renal phosphate reabsorption (Agus et al., 1971).

Unfortunately, it is not known what is the interaction between phosphate and calcium metabolism and specifically how phosphaturia affects calcium homeostasis. At one time this relationship was thought to be the key to the mechanism of action of the hormone (Albright and Reifenstein, 1948); this view is no longer accepted, but the relationship between phosphate metabolism and decreased renal phosphate reabsorption, on the one hand, and calcium homeostasis and metabolism, on the other, still requires qualitative and quantitative definition.

Calcitonin

The discovery of calcitonin (see Chapter 11), a hypocalcemic polypeptide produced by the C cells of the mammalian thyroid gland, at once raised the question of the function of this compound. It seemed logical to attribute to it an action opposite to that of parathyroid hormone. As will be shown, this turned out not to be the case. However, the approach outlined above for parathyroid hormone and based on a cybernetic analysis of calcium homeostasis proved useful for the study of the regulatory role of this hormone (Bronner *et al.*, 1967; Sammon *et al.*, 1969).

If calcitonin had a similar but opposite action to parathyroid hormone, one would have expected that removal of the cells producing this hormone would have both transient and steady-state effects on plasma calcium homeostasis. For example, one would expect that animals without this hormone would control their steady-state calcium less well than normal animals. At the same time, one would have predicted changes in both intensity and relative importance of bone calcium deposition and removal rates and/or of renal calcium reabsorption and filtration rates. On the basis of such changes one would then be able to analyze the regulatory role of this hormone in calcium homeostasis.

The results of such studies (Bronner *et al.*, 1967, 1968; Sammon *et al.*, 1969) may be summarized as follows: Calcitonin has no evident steady-state effect on calcium metabolism. Animals deprived of their endogenous supply of the hormone can regulate their plasma calcium as well as control animals. In other words, thyroidectomized animals supplied with *l*-thyroxine in the food and bearing functional parathyroid autografts (TCTX) do as well as euthyroid controls with functional parathyroid autografts (C), as far as steady-state plasma calcium control is concerned. This is shown by the following equations:

$$[Ca_s] = 10.04 + 0.007 \, S_i \quad \text{(C)} \tag{22}$$

$$[Ca_s] = 9.72 + 0.017 \, S_i \quad \text{(TCTX)} \tag{23}$$

(units: $[Ca_s]$ = mg Ca/100 ml plasma; S_i = mg Ca/day)

Equations (22) and (23) do not differ significantly.

Calcitonin also has no effect on the hierarchical relationship of bone and kidney, as can be seen by comparing Eqs. (24) and (25):

$$\Delta = -0.06 + 0.97 \, S_i \quad \text{(C)} \tag{24}$$

$$\Delta = +0.00 + 0.95 \, S_i \quad \text{(TCTX)} \tag{25}$$

Moreover, by analyzing Eqs. (26–29) it can be seen that calcitonin removal had little or no effect on either intensity or relative regulatory importance of v_{o+} and v_{o-}:

$$v_{o+} = 68.2 + 0.26\ S_i \quad \text{(C)} \tag{26}$$

$$v_{o-} = 68.8 - 0.71\ S_i \quad \text{(C)} \tag{27}$$

$$v_{o+} = 63.1 + 0.28\ S_i \quad \text{(TCTX)} \tag{28}$$

$$v_{o-} = 63.1 - 0.67\ S_i \quad \text{(TCTX)} \tag{29}$$

(units: mg Ca/day)

Bone calcium and phosphorus content also were similar in both groups.

It thus appears that calcitonin, in contrast with parathyroid hormone, has no effect on the steady-state regulation of plasma calcium. Loads that in parathyroidectomized animals induce significant steady-state errors—presumably because of altered function of the major controller, bone—fail to induce such errors in animals without an endogenous calcitonin supply. The latter indeed behave like normal animals.

However, when animals without an endogenous calcitonin supply are subjected to acute calcium-loading studies, it takes them appreciably longer to overcome this acute positive disturbance (Talmage *et al.*, 1965; Bronner *et al.*, 1967). The time course of their plasma calcium error is quite similar to that of surgically parathyroidectomized animals (Bronner *et al.*, 1968). Since measurements of plasma calcitonin levels have shown that above the normal reference calcium level calcitonin release varies positively and proportionately with plasma calcium (Care *et al.*, 1968), calcitonin would appear to play an acute regulatory role. In man-made systems the addition of a derivative control to a pre-existing proportional control provides a mechanism for faster error correction without the danger of overshoot (Goldman, 1960). The time-error curve of a derivative plus proportional control is similar to that of an integral plus proportional control. However, in a situation of integral plus proportional controls there is no steady-state error, while in a situation of derivative plus proportional controls a steady-state error exists.

On the basis of these considerations, Bronner *et al.* (1968) have proposed that calcitonin acts like a derivative, i.e., a transient and not a steady-state control.

If this is so, one would predict that steady-state calcium homeostasis would be the same in PTX and thyroparathyroidectomized (TPTX) animals, but that PTX animals would be able to overcome an acute load better than TPTX animals. Comparative studies on PTX and TPTX animals (Bronner *et al.*, 1968) indicate differences in acute error correction at high loads that, though small, are as predicted, i.e., somewhat faster error correction by the PTX as compared to the TPTX rats.

It is generally accepted that calcitonin acts exclusively via bone (Chapter 11; Copp, 1969). Therefore, the regulatory action of this hormone may be summarized as follows:

1. Calcitonin is released in proportion to the derivative of the positive error of the plasma calcium.

2. The released hormone acts on bone to inhibit calcium release into bone.

3. The effect of hormone action is a more precise control of the acute positive error of the plasma calcium. (No data have been published on the effect of negative error in animals deprived of endogenous calcitonin.)

These statements form the basis of the regulatory diagram shown in Fig. 11. It is similar to that depicted in Fig. 10, except for the addition of the action of calcitonin, which is shown to be released in response to the derivative of a positive plasma calcium error. Presumably, the action of calcitonin would lead to a temporary drop in v_{o-}, with no effect on v_{o+} (Milhaud *et al.*, 1965; O'Riordan and Aurbach, 1968). This would cause the plasma calcium to drop to its reference value, when calcitonin action would cease. Such a model predicts that hormone release would be slower the smaller the difference between the actual plasma calcium value and its reference level (for further theoretical analysis of the relationship between plasma calcitonin and calcium levels, see Bronner, 1973).

The physiological significance of the regulatory role played by calcitonin is difficult to understand (see also Chapter 11), since it is unclear how faster error correction by itself can benefit an organism. The physiological benefits derived from the presence of parathyroid hormone are not difficult to imagine. Higher rates of turnover tend to be

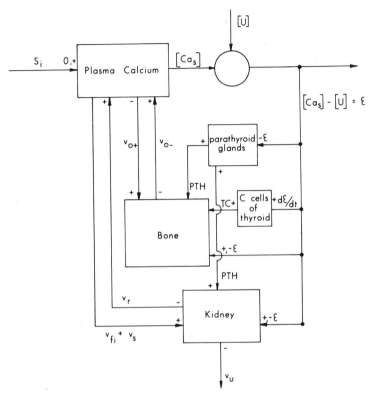

Fig. 11. Diagram of plasma calcium regulation including parathyroid hormone (PHT) and calcitonin (TC) action. For explanation of symbols, see legend of Fig. 10. S_i is the disturbing signal, v_{o+}, v_{o-}, v_r, v_{fi}, and v_s are the controlling signals, with bone and kidney responses proportional to either the positive or negative error, ϵ. The parathyroid glands respond to the negative error by release of parathyroid hormone, PTH, which acts on bone and kidney. The C cells of the thyroid gland respond to the derivative of the positive error by releasing calcitonin, TC, which acts on bone. Bone and kidney alone bring about proportional error correction. The addition of calcitonin action on bone is the equivalent of the addition of a derivative control which brings faster transient error correction. The addition of parathyroid hormone action on bone and kidney is the equivalent of the addition of an integral control that brings about faster negative error correction and virtually eliminates positive steady-state errors. (From Bronner, 1973, and reproduced by permission of the publisher.)

associated with larger structures and a larger skeleton may have evolutionary benefits. Moreover, since nearly all of the ingested calcium ends up in the skeleton, a system like the parathyroid glands that mobilizes calcium when the exogenous supply is temporarily limited is of obvious benefit. On the other hand, a sudden, harmful rise in the plasma calcium due to the ingestion of a dietary source unexpectedly rich in calcium seems improbable. In unpublished experiments (B. G. Shah, P. J. Sammon, and F. Bronner) it proved impossible significantly to raise the plasma calcium of animals without endogenous calcitonin beyond that of controls, even though both groups had been trained to eat their entire daily ration in half an hour. However, Gray and Munson (1969) were able to demonstrate differences in an experiment in which they administered calcium by gavage to control and experimental animals. In any event, both the mode of action and the physiological role of calcitonin seem subtle and as yet elusive. At present, calcitonin is indeed a hormone in search of a function.

Concluding Remarks

Kinetic anlysis has proved useful as a basis for cybernetic analysis. This in turn has led to better understanding of the roles of bone and kidney and how these are modified by parathyroid hormone and calcitonin. There are other aspects of regulation for which the concepts of kinetic analysis may prove quite useful. One is what is known as nutritional requirement. In terms of calcium this is generally defined as the amount needed to keep an adult individual in zero balance, i.e., to provide him enough intake so that his output equals his intake. In other words, his bodily calcium balance, Δ, equals zero. But since $\Delta = v_{o+} - v_{o-}$, one can imagine a situation when v_{o+} and v_{o-} are high and equal or low and equal. There is no reason to suppose, however, that rates of high and low turnover are necessarily physiologically equivalent. A patient with hyperparathyroidism has high rates of turnover and one with hypoparathyroidism has low rates of turnover. Both may be in zero balance, yet they are obviously not equivalent. Thus a calcium requirement based only on a measurement of Δ is not very revealing. One based on kinetic and/or cybernetic measurements is likely to be more meaningful.

Another problem where cybernetic analysis may help is with the role played by other hormones. Here the approach used for parathyroid hormone and calcitonin may serve as a model. Essentially one investigates the contribution toward homeostasis made by a given hormone under conditions of acute and chronic stress. For example, if a thyroidectomized animal were to be found to handle steady-state and acute calcium loads as well as a normal one, this would be presumptive evidence that thyroxin plays no role in calcium homeostasis; of course such a finding is unlikely in view of the studies by Krane et al. (1965).

Finally, the cybernetic approach may help differentiate between diseases of regulation and diseases in which the response is appropriate, but the eliciting signal is inappropriate. Contrast renal disease in which there is an enzymatic defect incapable of converting 25-hydroxycalciferol (25-HC) to 1,25-dihydroxycalciferol (1,25-DHC) with a disease in which there is a defect in the intestinal synthesis of nuclear binding protein for 1,25-dihydroxcalciferol [for purposes of this example it is assumed that parathyroid hormone (PTH) and 1,25-DHC are both needed in bone to permit normal bone turnover, but only 1,25-DHC (and not PTH) is needed in the intestine]. In the first case, where there is a renal enzymatic defect, there will be call for PTH and the patient will show evidence of secondary hyperparathyroidism. There will be depressed calcium absorption and, hypersecretion of PTH nothwithstanding, the plasma calcium will tend to be low. Yet there is no defect of regulation. In the second case, however, the inability to bind and dispose of 1,25-DHC will lead to a build-up of this compound, a tendency for high bone turnover, yet inadequate absorption, and a regulatory defect involving the complicated interaction between blood calcium, bone, PTH, and 1,25-DHC. A load study will reveal an absorptive defect and an apparent overresponse in terms of 1,25-DHC. This would be an example of a regulatory defect.

One could imagine another type of regulatory defect, one in which a positive feedback signal is generated and increased. The author is unaware of a disease situation that can rigorously be so described, though such an eventuality cannot of course be ruled out.

There is little question that compared to other systems (e.g., the cardiovascular, Guyton et al., 1972) calcium regulation is simple. It is therefore to be hoped that the present chapter will help attract further interest to and permit additional progress in this field.

Chapter 15

CELLULAR FUNCTIONS OF CALCIUM

GIDEON A. RODAN

This chapter deals with the functions of calcium other than in calcified tissues. Calcium plays an important role in many cellular functions, including nerve excitation, muscular contraction, mitochondria and cellular extrusion processes, to mention only some. The field is much too broad to permit exhaustive review in a single chapter. However, this volume would be incomplete without at least a brief discussion of some of the more important or more thoroughly studied calcium-dependent processes.

Calcium and Nerve Excitation

Pulse propagation along a nerve fiber, as studied primarily in the giant squid axon, is accompanied by a reversal of the resting potential (which measures about 50 mV, positive on the outside), to give rise to the action potential (around 110 mV, negative outside), soon thereafter followed by the restoration of the initial conditions (Hodgkin and Katz, 1949). These transmembrane potential changes have been shown to result from a transient redistribution of sodium and potassium which in turn is due to changes in the permeability of the membrane to these ions. Thus, the nerve membrane, which under resting conditions is permeable to potassium and relatively impermeable to sodium, becomes temporarily permeable to sodium and impermeable to potassium. This causes sodium to flow into the cell. At the peak of the action potential the permeability to potassium is again highly increased and the outflow of potassium accelerates the repolarization of the membrane and brings about restoration of the resting potential (Keynes, 1951; Keynes and Lewis, 1951; Hodgkin *et al.*, 1952; Hodgkin and Huxley, 1952; Hodgkin, 1951).

Calcium concentration in the ambient medium has been found to have a definite effect on these events. Phenomenologically, a reduction of the calcium concentration in the medium of the giant squid axon from 112 mM to 22 mM has the same effect as a reduction in the resting membrane potential by 10–15 mV. Thus, at the lower calcium concentrations the inward sodium current caused by depolarization (20–60 mV) of the nerve fiber is larger. The rate of rise and fall of the sodium conductance, caused by the appropriate electric stimuli, also increases when the calcium concentration is lowest. The potassium current (outward) also increases, as does the rate of rise of potassium conductance (under a cathode). At zero calcium concentration the nerve fiber slowly loses the ability to undergo changes in sodium and potassium conductance and assumes a refractory state, the potassium conductance remaining high and the sodium conductance inactivated. Traces of calcium are sufficient to allow limited changes in conductance to occur. Full function is rapidly restored when the calcium concentration is raised to normal levels (Frankenhaeuser and Hodgkin, 1957). These findings have been substantiated in the myelinated fiber of the frog sciatic nerve. There, too, the amplitude of the action potential is smaller at low calcium concentrations, the excitability is lost reversibly in a calcium-free medium, and small traces of calcium (< 0.01 mM) are sufficient to maintain excitability (Frankenhaeuser, 1957). Two hypotheses have been advanced to explain the mechanism of action of calcium:

(a) Calcium ions adsorbed to the membrane affect the distribution of charges inside the membrane and therefore its electrical stability.

(b) The removal of calcium unblocks sodium permeation sites ("carriers") and facilitates depolarization.

Neither hypothesis is entirely satisfactory to explain all results quanti-tatively (Frankenhaeuser and Hodgkin, 1957).

For a better understanding of its role in nerve excitation calcium ion movement was studied during pulse propagation (Hodgkin and Keynes, 1957). The calcium flux in the resting giant squid axon has been estimated, from radioisotope studies, at 0.1 pmole/cm²/second. Stimulation over a range of 50–156 impulses/second caused additional Ca to enter the axon at the rate of 0.006 pmole/cm²/impulse. When the calcium concentration in the medium was increased from 10.7 to 22 mM and magnesium was dropped from 55 mM to zero, influx in-creased to 0.4 pmole Ca/cm²/second under resting conditions and to 0.01 pmole/cm²/impulse when the nerve was stimulated. Raising the concentration to 112 mM increased calcium influx in the stimulated axon to 0.08 pmole/cm²/impulse. When the membrane was depolarized by raising the external potassium concentration, calcium influx in-creased to a lesser extent than when the nerve was stimulated electri-cally (156 impulses/second).

Calcium efflux from nerve is a slow process, with a half-life of about 20 hours, and is unaffected by axon stimulation. The reason for this may be that calcium enters the axon through the sodium channels. Once inside the nerve, further axonal movement of calcium appears quite small, suggesting that most axonal calcium is bound (Hodgkin and Keynes, 1957). These findings have recently received further sup-port from studies using aequorin as an indicator of ionic calcium con-centration. Aequorin is a jellyfish protein that emits light in the presence of ionized calcium. With the aid of this indicator it was shown that the ionized calcium concentration in the resting axon does not exceed 0.3 μM. Raising the external calcium concentration and/or stimulating the axon increased aequorin glow. After stimulation, the light emittance returned to the basal level, presumably because of calcium uptake by an internal calcium store (Baker et al., 1971). This possibility derives support from an earlier finding that about two hours after incubation with cyanide, calcium efflux from a resting axon increased 5–15-fold. This effect was reversed as soon as cyanide was removed. Cyanide also increased the dialyzable fraction of axoplasmic calcium. Since cyanide inhibits ATP formation it might cause the release of calcium from a cellular storage site endowed with an ATP-dependent mechanism for calcium accumulation—presumably the mitochondrion. The extrusion of this liberated calcium against a concentration gradient, when most of the ATP has been broken down, can be explained as resulting from the coupling of calcium efflux to sodium influx (Blaustein and Hodgkin, 1969). This explanation is based on the observation that the cyanide effect is reduced when the external calcium is replaced by magnesium, or sodium by lithium. Calcium extrusion is insensitive to ouabain, a glycoside that inhibits the Na^+-, K^+-, Mg-dependent ATPase, an enzyme considered to be involved in active sodium transport. Coupling of sodium to calcium transport in the opposite direction has been proposed by Baker et al. (1969). They recorded a small component of sodium efflux that is calcium dependent, insensitive to ouabain, and is abolished by cyanide. A sodium-dependent calcium influx has also been reported. It increased when the external sodium concentration was reduced and the sodium efflux enhanced. The entry of 1 calcium ion is thought to be coupled to the exit of about 3 sodium ions (Baker et al., 1971). Both calcium efflux from cyanide-poisoned and unpoisoned axons and calcium-dependent sodium efflux have been found to have a Q_{10} of 2–3.

The aequorin studies have also shown that there are two phases to the entry of calcium into the giant squid axon during depolarization. The early phase is abolished by tetrodotoxin, an inhibitor of sodium conductance, and is assumed to take place through the sodium channels. The late phase, occurring during the potassium conductance, is not impaired by its inhibitor tetraethylammonium and has similar characteristics to the calcium entry responsible for the release of neural transmitter at the presynaptic nerve terminals (Baker et al., 1971).

Calcium in Neuromuscular and Synaptic Transmission

It has been known for over 30 years that the transmission of the nerve impulse to the muscle fiber is mediated by the neural transmitter acetyl choline. Released by quantal discharges (Fatt and Katz, 1952) from the nerve ending of the neuromuscular junction, acetyl choline moves to the end plate of the muscle fiber. There, acetyl choline causes an increase in ion permeability (Takeuchi and Takeuchi, 1960), which in turn generates the end plate potential, the electrical stimulus leading to muscle contraction.

The critical role of the calcium ion in the first part of the process was demonstrated by a very elegant experiment (Katz and Miledi, 1965). A micropipette filled with calcium was introduced into the neuromuscular junction of a frog sartorius preparation immersed in a calcium-free medium. The excitation of the nerve produced no junction potential unless some calcium was flowed through the micropipette at the same time.

The temporal relationship between the neural pulse and the requirement for calcium has been studied in detail by Katz and Miledi (1967a,b). These workers found that calcium has to be applied either before or during depolarization of the nerve ending in order for acetyl choline release to occur several milliseconds later; this indicates that calcium plays a specific role in the process of acetyl choline secretion.

The quantitative aspects of the calcium requirement have also been studied. The relationship between calcium concentration and the number of acetyl choline quanta released fits a model according to which about 4 calcium ions, acting cooperatively, are required to bring about the release of 1 quantum of acetyl choline (Dodge et al., 1969).

Several other ions can replace, inhibit or facilitate the effect of calcium. A reduction in external sodium concentration increases the quantal output of acetyl choline (Kelly, 1965). This has been explained to be due to competition between sodium and calcium for the same binding sites at the nerve ending (Colomo and Rahamimoff, 1968). Intracellular sodium, however, increases the number of quanta released (Birks and Cohen, 1968a,b) and the explanation offered was that intracellular sodium enhances calcium influx (Baker et al., 1969). Magnesium (Hubbard et al., 1968), as well as manganese and beryllium (Blioch et al., 1968), inhibits the action of calcium, presumably by competing for a common binding site (Hubbard et al., 1968). Strontium and barium can replace calcium (Miledi, 1966), but are less effective (Dodge et al., 1969). Calcium, however, is the only physiological agent that permits transmitter release to occur following nerve depolarization (Katz and Miledi, 1969a; 1970). The model for the mechanism of calcium action is conjectural at this stage. Nerve depolarization increases the permeability of the axon membrane to calcium; this in turn results in increased calcium influx. One model assumes that this calcium is required for the fusion of acetyl choline-containing vesicles with the axon membrane, followed eventually by the quantal discharge of the vesicular content (Katz, 1971).

This scheme is analogous to the release of neurotransmitter substances in other nerve synapses. Electron microscopy has indeed revealed the existence of clusters of synaptic vesicles near the presynaptic release sites (deRobertis and Bennet, 1954; Palade and Palay, 1954).

Both the electrophysiological properties of nerve synapses and their sensitivity to different ions are similar to those of the neuromuscular junction, in all of which calcium plays a central role. In experiments on the giant synapse of the squid measurement of the ratio between the postsynaptic and the presynaptic potentials made it possible to single out the effects of calcium on synaptic transmission from its general effect on nerve depolarization (Katz and Miledi 1967c). This ratio was found to increase with calcium concentration. Quantitative studies showed that this increase is roughly proportional to the square of the calcium concentration; this suggests that at least 2 calcium ions are required for the release of 1 quantum of transmitter (Katz and Miledi, 1970). Magnesium and manganese have been found to depress the postsynaptic response (Katz and Miledi, 1967c), whereas strontium and barium are able, in part, to replace calcium (Katz and Miledi, 1969b).

Essentially, the involvement of calcium in synaptic transmission, including the neuromuscular synapse, is considered to be similar to that in cellular extrusion processes in general. These will be dealt with in more detail below.

Calcium and Cellular Extrusion Processes

The requirement for calcium in neuromuscular transmission has now been recognized as an example of what seems to be a general biological phenomenon. Evidence accumulated during recent years indicates that calcium ions are essential for the occurrence of secretion in response to specific stimuli, in practically all instances where cellular secretion takes place.

The best documented case is the secretion of catecholamines from the chromaffin cells of the adrenal medulla in response to acetyl choline stimulation. It was shown about 10 years ago that if feline

(Douglas and Rubin, 1961) or bovine (Philippu and Schümann, 1962) adrenal glands are perfused with acetylcholine, or its substitute, carbachol, catecholamin secretion does not occur in the absence of calcium. It has also been shown that for a given dose of acetylcholine the secretory response increases with calcium concentration (Douglas and Rubin, 1961) and that there is no requirement for sodium and potassium (Douglas and Rubin, 1963). Magnesium inhibits secretion, whereas barium and strontium can substitute for calcium (Douglas and Rubin, 1964). Acetylcholine stimulation enhances the influx of calcium into chromaffin cells (Douglas and Poisner, 1962) and tetracaine and magnesium, both inhibitors of catecholamine secretion, inhibit calcium uptake (Rubin et al., 1967). It was therefore concluded that calcium influx is the event that couples stimulation to secretion.

Calcium penetration has been assumed to occur as a result of increased membrane permeability which results from depolarization caused by acetylcholine (Douglas, 1968). The mechanism of calcium influx has not yet been totally clarified, but it seems that secretion varies directly with the extent of depolarization and with the calcium level in the ambient medium. This suggests that calcium influx is a passive process. It appears, however, that as in the case of the giant squid axon (Baker et al., 1969), calcium influx may depend on the intracellular sodium concentration. Thus when adrenal glands were perfused with ouabain, which inhibits the Na^+K^+-ATPase and increases the intracellular sodium concentration, an enhanced response to acetylcholine was observed (Banks, 1967). A decrease in intracellular potassium concentration, resulting from perfusion with potassium-free medium, had a similar effect (Banks et al., 1969). On the other hand, prolonged perfusion with sodium-free solutions inhibits the secretory response, presumably by decreasing the intracellular sodium concentration. This inhibition can be overcome by raising the calcium concentration in the medium (Banks et al., 1969). These facts are compatible with the view that calcium influx is inversely related to the intracellular sodium concentration.

An interesting aspect of calcium translocation during acetylcholine stimulation of the chromaffin cells is the concentration of the ion within the catecholamine-containing granules (Borowitz, 1969). These granules have been shown to contain an ATP–magnesium-dependent catecholamine pump (Taugner and Hasselbach, 1966), with some of

→the features of the calcium pump found in muscle. It was therefore suggested that the granules control the intracellular calcium concentration in a way similar to the sarcoplasmic reticulum of the muscle.

The actual process by which calcium participates in catecholamine secretion is not yet understood. By itself calcium does not stimulate secretion from isolated chromaffin granules, whereas ATP does (Poisner and Trifaro, 1967). The metabolism of the intact gland must be normal in order for calcium to manifest its secretory action (Rubin, 1969, 1970a). An analogy has been drawn between the role of calcium in cellular secretion and in muscular contraction (Douglas, 1968; Rubin, 1970a). We shall return to the details of this model after first listing a few other calcium-requiring secretory systems.

Neurohypophyseal secretion of vasopressin and oxytocin bears a relationship to calcium that is similar to that of catecholamine secretion, calcium being required for secretion to occur in response to the appropriate stimuls (Ishida, 1967, 1968). The level of secretion is directly related to the calcium concentration in the medium (Douglas and Poisner, 1964a) and radiocalcium exchange is enhanced during stimulation of the neurohypophysis (Douglas and Poisner, 1964b). Barium can replace calcium and also enhances vasopressin secretion when added to a solution containing calcium (Haller et al., 1965). Magnesium and sodium are inhibitory (Douglas and Poisner, 1964a). As in the case of catecholamine secretion from chromaffin cells, oxytocin and vasopressin secretion are stimulated by ouabain (Dicker, 1966).

The feature common to neuromuscular and nerve synapses, on the one hand, and to the adrenal and posterior pituitary cells, on the other, is that all are either part of or are developmentally related to the nervous system, and membrane depolarization is an intermediate step in the events that lead from stimulation to secretion.

Calcium, however, also appears essential to the secretions of the adenohypophysis which is considered to be of nonnervous origin. Thus, the secretion of ACTH (Kraicer et al., 1969), prolactin (Parsons, 1969), luteinizing hormone (Samli and Geschwind, 1968), and thyrotropin (Vale et al., 1967), all seem to require calcium in a way similar to that described above.

A special case is that of thyrocalcitonin and parathyroid hormone, endocrine secretions that have been dealt with in detail earlier in

Chapter 11. For these hormones, which participate directly in calcium metabolism, the plasma calcium concentration itself is the stimulus for release.

Another well-documented case of the calcium requirement for endocrine secretion is that of insulin. Release of this polypeptide occurs in response to glucose, tolbutamide, and other agents and is proportional to the calcium level (Curry et al., 1968). Barium can substitute for calcium while magnesium inhibits insulin secretion (Hales and Milner, 1968). Sodium affects insulin release in a way similar to its effect on adrenal secretion. Thus ouabain and potassium deprivation, both of which cause sodium accumulation in the β-cells, stimulate insulin secretion (Hales and Milner, 1968).

In the case of the exocrine glands, there is evidence to suggest that calcium is involved in the complex secretions of the salivary glands. In perfused glands secretion of water and protein in response to acetyl choline and noradrenaline stimulation varies directly with calcium concentration (Douglas and Poisner, 1963; Peterson et al., 1967). Sympathetic and parasympathetic agents greatly increase calcium fluxes in the rat salivary gland (Dreisbach, 1964). Because these effects are inhibited by metabolic inhibitors, calcium uptake may involve active transport. Indeed, an ATP-dependent "calcium pump" has been shown to be present in the microsomal fractions of rat parotid and submaxillary glands (Selinger et al., 1970).

The amylase secretion by the exocrine pancreas has also been shown to be dependent on the presence of calcium (Hokin, 1966).

Other calcium-dependent cellular extrusion processes are the protein secretions from polymorphonuclear leukocytes and the secretion of HCl from the gastric mucosa. Staphylococcal leucocidin-induced excretion of enzymes (β-glucosidase, ribonuclease, peroxidase) from rabbit polymorphonuclear leukocytes is accompanied by potassium efflux (Woodin and Wieneke, 1968) and requires calcium in the medium (Woodin and Wieneke, 1963, 1964, 1970). Another interesting feature is that the addition of the energy-rich phosphonucleotides, ADP and ATP, to the medium enhances the ability of calcium to induce secretion after prolonged incubation in calcium-free medium (Woodin and Wieneke, 1963).

The gastric secretion of HCl has been shown to be related directly to the calcium concentration of the plasma (Barreras and Donaldson,

1967) or of the *in vitro* incubation medium of gastric mucosa (Jacobson *et al.*, 1965; Schwartz *et al.*, 1967). Calcium appears to be localized within the granules of the mucosal cells. These granules tend to disappear in a calcium-free medium (Schwartz *et al.*, 1967). Again this is evidence that calcium is required for the release of substances from intracellular vesicles.

Histamine is secreted from mast cells or leukocytes as a result of the antigen–antibody reaction. This secretion is also inhibited by calcium deprivation (Mongar and Schild, 1962), as is histamine secretion induced by antiserum. Histamine release in response to certain organic bases (like compound 48/80) proceeds, however, in the absence of calcium (Saeki, 1964). ATP also causes histamine release from mast cells; its action is dependent upon calcium and is inhibited by magnesium (Diamant and Krüger, 1967). During the process ATP is split by an ATPase (Diamant, 1967) and inhibition of the splitting enzyme inhibits histamine release.

Finally, mention should be made of the calcium-dependent cellular secretion of serotonin. This vasoconstrictor compound is secreted from thrombocytes in the presence of thrombin (Grette, 1962) or antigen (Humphrey and Jaques, 1955). Secretion does not occur when a calcium-chelating agent is added to the medium and is restored upon the addition of calcium (Markwardt and Barthel, 1964; Markwardt *et al.*, 1965). Calcium also enhances the spontaneous release of serotonin from isolated thrombocyte granules (Pletscher *et al.*, 1968).

There are basically two hypotheses, not mutually exclusive, that attempt to explain the role of calcium in cellular extrusion processes.

The first originated from the electron microscopic observation (Palade and Palay, 1954) that secretory cells store secreta within granules that eventually fuse with the cell wall and thereby release their contents. In support of this hypothesis is the observation that during secretion the granular contents can be detected in the medium (Kirschner *et al.*, 1967), but not so cell plasma proteins or granular wall lipoids (Schneider *et al.*, 1967; Kirschner *et al.*, 1967). It has also been shown that empty granules remain in the cells after stimulation (Mahamed *et al.*, 1968). Calcium has been assumed to serve as an ionic bridge essential for the fusion of the granules to the cell wall membranes. To reach the cell wall, the granules have to travel through the cellular cytoplasm and overcome the potential barrier of the membrane charge. Making a number of assumptions, Mathews (1970) has calculated that the kinetic energy of random movement would be sufficient to bring the granules close enough to the cell wall, where higher calcium concentrations would prevail following membrane depolarization.

Since secretion has been shown to require metablic energy, usually provided by the splitting of ATP (Rubin, 1969, 1970a,b), the second hypothesis draws an analogy between the role calcium plays in the coupling of excitation to muscular contraction via membrane depolarization and the coupling of secretory stimuli to secretion (Douglas, 1968). The analogy is based on the fact that secretion, like muscular contraction, has been shown to require metabolic energy, usually provided by the splitting of ATP (Rubin, 1969, 1970a,b). The discrete steps and subcellular structures involved in the series of events leading from stimulation and ATP splitting to mechanical extrusion of the secreted substance remain to be identified, as does the locus of calcium action. Perhaps microtubules and microfilaments, found in many cells, may be related to the process of cellular extrusion as agents of intracellular locomotion, requiring calcium for contraction.

The Role of Calcium in Muscular Contraction

The investigation of the mechanism of muscular contraction represents one of the most successful phases in molecular physiology. It is now generally accepted that the control of muscular contraction and relaxation is mediated by the concentration of calcium in the sarcoplasm, which in turn is regulated by the sarcoplasmic reticulum. The subject has been thoroughly and comprehensively reviewed (Ebashi and Endo, 1968; Martonosi, 1971) and will be covered here only in broad outline.

Since the classic work of Szent-Györgyi (1951) it has been known that muscular contraction is the result of the coupled activity of two muscular proteins, actin and myosin, requiring the presence of Mg, ATP and Ca. The actomyosin complex possesses ATPase activity. The splitting of ATP provides the energy needed to bring about a conformational change of the muscle proteins, which is the molecular event underlying the transition of the muscle fibril from the relaxed to the contracted state. This process depends on several factors including ionic strength, temperature and pH, but calcium is now recognized to be the central regulator of the contraction–relaxation cycle. In 1954 it was found that EDTA in the presence of ATP induced relaxation of glycerinated fibers (Bozler, 1954; Watanabe, 1955) in a way similar to the "muscle extract" discovered earlier (Marsh, 1951, 1952; Bendall, 1952, 1953; Fujita, 1954). In 1959 Weber pointed out that the actomyosin ATPase activity was dependent on the concentration of ionic calcium (Weber, 1959), and in 1960 Ebashi showed that the relaxing activity of different chelating agents was proportional to their calcium-binding capacity (Ebashi, 1960). At the same time it was demonstrated that the relaxing factor extracted from muscle was capable of accumulating calcium in the presence of ATP (Ebashi, 1960, 1961a,b; Ebashi and Lipmann, 1962; Hasselbach and Makinose, 1961). The structure of the relaxing factor was identified by electron microscopy as part of the sarcoplasmic reticulum (Nagai et al., 1960; Porter, 1961). Anatomically, the T system consists of invaginations of the outer membrane of the sarcolemma, ending with the triads and diads, which are special regions of interaction of the T-system membrane with the sacs of the sarcoplasmic reticulum. The latter is a membrane-enclosed subcellular structure, analogous to the endoplasmic reticulum of other tissues. It had already been shown that the central tubules of the triads convey the electrical stimulus from the sarcolemma to the interior of the cell (Huxley and Taylor, 1955, 1958). A general model thus emerged according to which depolarization of the sarcoplasmic reticulum causes calcium release. This activates the actomyosin ATPase, brings about muscular contraction, and is followed by an ATP-dependent reaccumulation of calcium in the sarcoplasmic reticulum leading to muscular relaxation (Ebashi, 1961a,b,c; Heilbrunn and Wiercinski, 1947, Niedergerke, 1955; Weber and Herz, 1963, 1964; Weber et al., 1963; Seidel and Gergely, 1963). Ample evidence has now accumulated supporting this scheme and also partly unveiling the mechanisms of the different steps involved. Some of this evidence will be presented in the order in which the events occur in the course of muscular contraction and relaxation.

The experiments of A. F. Huxley and co-workers (Huxley and Taylor, 1955, 1958; Huxley and Straub, 1958; Huxley and Peachey, 1964) have shown that the spread of the depolarization wave through the internal membrane system of the diad or triad (Porter and Palade, 1957) is the first in a series of events linking excitation to contraction. The continuity of the extracellular space with the intracellular T system has been convincingly demonstrated by a variety of methods (Franzini-Armstrong and Porter, 1964; H. E. Huxley, 1964; Page, 1965; Hill, 1964; Endo, 1964; Smith, 1966; Simpson and Oertelis, 1961; Simpson, 1965; Forssmann and Girardier, 1970; Jasper, 1967; Bertaud et al., 1970). Estimates of the capacitance of muscle fibers have also indicated that the T tubules and the external membrane are part of the same membrane system (Falk and Fatt, 1964; Gage and Eisenberg, 1969). All of this implies that the action potential generated at the myoneural junction would lead to the depolarization of the internal membrane down to the level of the triads, where the coupling of excitation to contraction presumably occurs. The coupling materializes through an increase in the concentration of the free calcium in the sarcoplasm. This can be demonstrated by a calcium-binding dye (Jöbsis and O'Connor, 1966) and by the inhibitory effect of injected EGTA,* a specific calcium binder (Hagiwara and Nakajima, 1966). The source of this calcium and the mechanism of its release are not yet fully known. There is evidence to indicate that calcium is stored in the terminal cysternae of the sarcoplasmic reticulum (Hasselbach, 1964a; Pease et al., 1965; Constantin et al., 1965). Its release is due to changes in membrane permeability caused either by depolarization (Constantin and Podolsky, 1966) or by a chemical transmitter which is secreted at the surface of the T system and diffuses to the membrane of the sarcoplasmic reticulum. The fine structure of the junctional area revealed by recent electron microscopic studies (Franzinin-Armstrong, 1970, 1971; Bertaud et al., 1970, Kelly, 1969) supports the latter hypothesis.

The next step is the activation of the contraction mechanism by an increase in the calcium concentration. It is generally accepted that the essential mechanism of muscle contraction involves the interaction of myosin and actin in the presence of ATP. Earlier work had already shown that calcium is essential for contraction to occur (Szent-Györgyi, 1951). However, the susceptibility to calcium depends on the preparation of the muscle proteins. Perry and Grey (1956) have observed that EDTA depresses the ATPase activity of a "natural" actomyosin prep-

*EGTA, 1,2-bis(2-dicarboxymethylaminoethoxy)ethane.

aration, but not of a "synthetic" one. Moreover, a protein was extracted from muscle (Ebashi and Ebashi, 1964) which restored responsiveness to calcium when added to "synthetic" actomysin. This protein was similar to the tropomysin prepared by Bailey (1946, 1948; Bailey *et al.*, 1948), later designated as "native" tropomyosin. Purer preparations of tropomyosin did not exhibit the same properties. Eventually, an additional protein of globular nature was found, namely, troponin, which endows the purer tropomyosin with the properties of the native one, including its susceptibility to calcium control (Ebashi and Kodama, 1965, 1966). Presumably, native tropomyosin is composed of 2 molecules of tropomyosin and 1 of troponin (Ebashi and Endo, 1968). The effects of the reassembled complex on the physicochemical properties of F-actin (the actin filaments) are similar to those of native tropomyosin. Both preparations bind to F-actin (Ebashi and Kodama, 1966). Since troponin itself does not bind to F-actin, it may exert its effect via changes in the tropomyosin molecule. Troponin also seems to be the molecule that mediates the regulating action of calcium. It binds about 5 moles Ca/100,000 g with a binding constant of about $6 \times 10^5 M^{-1}$ (Ebashi *et al.*, 1967). A large part of the calcium bound to troponin is readily exchangeable. Tropomyosin does not bind calcium and the calcium bound to actin is not exchangeable. Myosin binds about 1 mole Ca/200,000 g, and the exchangeable part of it has a binding constant of $10^5 M^{-1}$ (Hasselbach, 1957, 1964b; Kitagawa *et al.*, 1961). In addition to its calcium-binding properties, troponin was proposed as the site of calcium regulation on the basis of the parallelism between the sensitivity of cardiac muscle to strontium and the affinity of cardiac troponin to the same ion (Ebashi *et al.*, 1967).

Thus, according to this model, calcium ions released from the sarcoplasmic reticulum bind to troponin and cause conformational changes which, via tropomyosin, activate F-actin. This makes it possible for the latter to interact with myosin to split ATP and to bring about contraction. Inversely, reduction in calcium concentration causes relaxation by a reversal of that sequence of events. This model, however, cannot account for all the observations, and the least clarified aspect of it relates to the actual mechanism of action of the calcium ion. Troponin has been found to be a mixture of several proteins (Hartshorne and Mueller, 1968; Greaser and Gergely, 1971) and its localization relative to the other muscle proteins makes it difficult to explain the movement of myosin crossbridges which are relatively far away from it (H. E. Huxley, 1971). On the other hand, there is evidence to show that calcium regulating contraction binds directly to myosin (Dancker, 1970; Lehman, et al., 1970). In insect fibrillar muscle a calcium-activated movement of crossbridges was observed in the absence of ATPase activity, suggesting a direct effect of calcium on myosin rather than through ATPase activation (Miller and Tregear, 1970). It is, however, well established that calcium stimulates muscular contraction and that relaxation is caused by a drop in calcium concentration. The stimulus for calcium uptake by the sarcoplasmic reticulum is supposed to be the late effect of the depolarization wave that causes calcium release (Ebashi and Endo, 1968), but the exact mode of initiating this step is yet to be clarified.

A great deal more is known about the mechanism of calcium uptake by the sarcoplasmic reticulum. This subject has been thoroughly studied and has recently been reviewed in detail (Martonosi, 1971). More than 10 years ago it was shown that the accumulation of calcium in the sarcoplasmic reticulum is an energy-requiring process, accompanied by the Mg-dependent hydrolysis of ATP (Ebashi, 1960, 1961; Ebashi and Lipmann, 1962; Hasselbach and Makinose, 1961, 1963; Makinose and Hasselbach, 1965). A constant relationship of 2 calcium atoms/mole ATP suggested that the two processes are coupled (Weber et al., 1966), but more recent evidence indicates that the Ca/ATP ratios are higher (Sreter, 1969; Baskin, 1971) and that calcium activation of ATPase occurs in the absence of calcium transport (Martonosi et al., 1968; Weber, 1971a,b). Calcium efflux from the sarcoplasmic reticulum particles induced by the presence of ADP, P_i, and extremely low calcium concentration in the medium is accompanied by the synthesis of ATP to the extent of 1 mole/2 calcium ions (Makinose and Hasselbach, 1971). This process also requires the presence of magnesium and seems to be the reverse of calcium uptake, mediated by the same carrier.

ATP is not a specific energy source. It can be replaced by other phosphorylated nucleotides as well as by acetyl phosphate, carbamyl phosphate, and p-nitrophenylphosphate (see Martonosi, 1971). In all cases the same mechanism is thought to be involved.

The cardinal feature of this ATPase (or phosphatase) is its activation by calcium ions. The calcium-sensitive step is assumed to be the formation of a phosphoprotein intermediate (Makinose, 1969; Yamamoto and Tonomura, 1967, 1968; Martonosi, 1967, 1969) that involves the binding of ATP, followed by the binding of Ca and the release of ADP. This process occurs on the outside of the membrane surface. The transport of calcium to the inside of the membrane involves a conformational change of a calcium-carrying phosphorylated protein. This event is followed by the release of calcium on the inside of the membrane, dephosphorylation, and return to the initial state. The microsomal membrane is relatively impermeable to calcium, but highly permeable to anions. It is not yet known to what extent calcium binds to inside components of the membrane and to what extent it is neutralized or precipitated by the freely diffusible anions (Carvalho, 1966, 1968a,b; Vanderkooi and Martonosi, 1971a,b). The presence of oxalate, phosphate, pyrophosphate, or fluoride enhances calcium transport (Martonosi and Feretos, 1964).

Another important requirement for the energy-dependent calcium transport is the presence of phospholipids in the membrane preparation (see Martonosi, 1971). Treatment with phospholipase C inhibits both ATPase activity and calcium transport. Partial activity can be restored by addition of lecithin, lysolecithin, or synthetic detergents (Martonosi *et al.*, 1968). The phospholipid-dependent step seems to involve the decomposition of the phosphoprotein intermediate.

Such are the general features of this finely tuned calcium pump, controlling a highly specialized process for linking excitation to muscular contraction. Similar processes are now being discovered in other tissues where calcium has a regulatory function.

Calcium and Mitochondria

In 1949 Lehninger had shown that Ca^{2+} uncouples oxidative phosphorylation in mitochondria and several years later it was found that Ca^{2+} stimulates mitochondrial respiration (Siekevitz and Potter, 1955), if the system is free of ATP or ADP. However, it remained for Vasington and Murphy (1961, 1962) and DeLuca and Engstrom (1961) to show that isolated mitochondria can accumulate massive quantities of calcium by an energy-dependent process. In these experiments calcium uptake was studied in the presence of ATP (or ADP), Mg, and phosphate and found to depend on electron transport, since the addition of electron transport-uncoupling agents, including 2,4-dinitrophenol, prevented calcium uptake.

It was later shown that calcium accumulation can also be supported by ATP hydrolysis (Rossi and Lehninger, 1963), which in turn is stimulated by the presence of calcium. This suggested a coupled reaction (Brierley *et al.*, 1964). The ATP-supported calcium uptake is also inhibited by oligomycin (Brierley *et al.*, 1964). The emerging picture is an energy-dependent calcium accumulation driven either by electron transport provided by respiration, or by ATP hydrolysis. Calcium transport is the favored process in the utilization of energy provided by respiration and has priority over oxidative phosphorylation (Rossi and Legninger, 1964). On the other hand, calcium stimulated both respiration and ATP hydrolysis in what appeared to be a stoichiometric relationship, identical to that observed during calcium accumulation. This was interpreted to indicate that the ion transport is chemically coupled to the energy source through a nonphosphorylated, high-energy intermediate (reviewed by Lehninger *et al.*, 1967).

Another important observation is that in the course of calcium uptake the medium becomes acid and the mitochondria alkaline. Studies by many investigators (Chappell *et al.*, 1965; Engstrom and DeLuca, 1963; Chance, 1965; Drahota *et al.*, 1965; Rasmussen *et al.*, 1965; Rossi *et al.*, 1966; Mitchell and Moyle, 1965a,b; Wenner, 1966; Snoswell, 1966) have shown that in the absence of permeant ions, like phosphate or acetate, the normally H^+-impermeable mitochondrial membrane ejects one proton (H^+) for each Ca^{2+} ion accumulated, in the same kind of electron transport-dependent process described above. The ratio of H^+ to Ca^{2+} was, however, found to vary. At low K^+ concentration 1 H^+ ion/Ca^{2+} ion would be ejected, but in the presence of high K^+ concentrations 2 H^+ would be ejected/Ca^{2+}, fully maintaining electroneutrality (Lehninger *et al.*, 1967; Rossi *et al.*, 1966). To incorporate proton ejection into the transport model assuming a high-energy intermediate it was postulated that the latter is protonated and acts as a $Ca^{2+}/2H^+$ exchange pump (Rasmussen *et al.*, 1965).

An alternate view, elaborated mainly by Mitchell (Mitchell and Moyle, 1965a,b; Mitchell, 1966) is known as the chemiosmotic hypothesis. Briefly stated it proposes that the electron transport, driven by

the respiratory chain, produces an H^+ gradient across the mitochondrial membrane by a vector-type arrangement. This in turn supplies the pull for oxidative phosphorylation or ion transport. Although
the validity of this model has not yet been fully proved, it is supported
by much of the evidence (Lehninger, 1970; Selwyn et al., 1970). The
high-energy intermediate acting as a calcium carrier is incompatible
with data showing a nonstoichiometric relation between calcium accumulation and electron transport (reviewed by Lehninger et al., 1967;
Lehninger, 1970). The calcium carrier would therefore be a calcium-
binding moiety, capable of transporting calcium in either direction,
depending on the electrochemical gradient. Such a carrier could be
either neutral, and carry a charge-compensating counterion, or it
could be electrogenic. In that case it could also be driven by an electrical gradient, as proposed by the chemiosmotic hypothesis. This
carrier would be independent of the respiratory chain (Lehninger,
1970; Chance and Azzi, 1969). Mitochondria were reported to have
two groups of calcium-binding sites, one with a very high affinity constant ($K_m = 0.1-1.0 \ \mu M$) (Reynfarje and Lehninger, 1969). It has been
suggested that the high affinity site may be part of a calcium carrier.
Recently calcium-binding proteins have been partly isolated from
mitochondria (Sottocasa et al., 1972; Gomez-Puyou et al., 1972) but
their relation to the mitochondrial calcium transport is only conjectural at this stage.

The form and the location of the intramitochondrial calcium vary
with the loading conditions. In the presence of phosphate enormous
amounts of calcium (2.5 μmole/mg protein) can be accumulated in the
mitochondria in the form of a calcium phosphate precipitate if ATP
or ADP and Mg^{2+} are also present (Lehninger et al., 1967; Leblanc
et al., 1970). The Ca^{2+}/P_i ratio is about 1.7 and the granular deposits
revealed by electron microscopy do not show the typical diffraction
pattern of hydroxyapatite (Lehninger, 1970). Other permeant anions,
like acetate, may also accompany calcium accumulation, but because
of the high solubility of calcium acetate, calcium uptake in the presence of acetate results in considerable swelling of the mitochondria.

The release or efflux of calcium from mitochondria appears to occur
through a reverse of the calcium uptake process rather than by passive
diffusion. Calcium efflux is enhanced by uncoupling agents and is accompanied by H^+ uptake. The direction of the calcium movement may

be controlled by factors other than calcium concentration. Lee *et al.*
(1971) have shown that the addition of a "cytoplasmic metabolic
factor" stimulates energy-coupled calcium uptake under conditions
under which it would not occur otherwise.

The physiological role of calcium accumulation in the mitochondria
is still being debated. The high affinity and capacity of the mitochondria
for calcium and the preference for calcium uptake over oxidative
phosphorylation would suggest that it plays an essential role in some
physiological function. Two processes have been considered in that
respect: the excitation–relaxation cycle of muscle (Patriarca and
Carafoli, 1969) and biological calcification (Lehninger, 1970), but present evidence is insufficient to prove direct mitochondrial involvement
in either of these processes.

Other Functions of Calcium and Concluding Remarks

The list of cellular and subcellular functions of calcium described
in the preceding sections is bound to be incomplete as it includes only
those examples where experimental evidence has elucidated, at
least in part, the mechanism of calcium involvement. Other functions
of calcium include its role in blood clotting, a function of calcium that
has been known and studied for many years. Calcium is also a constituent of cell membranes essential for cell adhesion and intercellular
junctional membrane permeability (Loewenstein, 1967a,b). Effects of
calcium on certain enzymes or enzyme systems have been reported,
although not as an obligatory component of the enzyme as is the case
in typical metalloenzymes. Calcium is involved in the regulation of
calcium-susceptible ATPases, activation of phosphorylase b kinase,
an enzyme essential in glycogenolysis (Ozawa *et al.*, 1967), activation of
certain adenyl cyclases (Bradham *et al.*, 1970; Lefkowitz *et al.*, 1970),
also modulation of metabolic pathways like renal gluconeogenesis
(Nagata and Rasmussen, 1970), among others. Calcium has been reported to stimulate catecholamine synthesis in the striatum of rats
(Goldstein *et al.*, 1970), protein synthesis in the adrenal of rats (Farese,
1971), as well as hemopoietic cell proliferation (Perris *et al.*, 1967). This
list, by no means exhausted, merely illustrates the wide variety of biological processes involving calcium. Common to all biological functions

of calcium is the effect of the ion on macromolecular tertiary structure, a result of the charge density on the ion surface.

From the point of view of the dynamics of biological processes one can distinguish two types of functions for the calcium ion: (a) Calcium serves as a stable structural component of macromolecular aggregates; and (b) calcium is a catalyst in a dynamic process. The role of calcium in stabilizing membrane structure or fibrin belongs to the first category. The role of calcium in muscular contraction or cellular secretion is an example of the second. To permit dynamic regulation the change in calcium concentration ought to be controlled by specific stimuli. Specialized structures have therefore evolved, capable of handling large calcium fluxes according to the functional requirements of the cell or tissue. The sarcoplasmic reticulum of the muscle is an example of a specialized organelle with the required organization to respond to the nerve-mediated stimulus by an energy-dependent calcium flux. Similar structures will probably be found in other systems where regulation is mediated by fluctuations in calcium concentration.

On the whole, regulation of biological processes by ions is a fascinating illustration of how the intricate biological organization can be coordinated by small and simple chemical entities that can move along a nonspecific electrical potential. This is, of course, made possible by the information "stored" in the ion-receptor sites of the macromolecules.

BIBLIOGRAPHY

Abramow, M., and Corvilain, J. (1967). *Nature (London)* **213**, 85.

Acheson, R. M. (1959). *J. Anat.* **93**, 123.

Adams, T. H., and Norman, A. W. (1970). *J. Biol. Chem.* **245**, 4421.

Adams, T. H., Wong, R. G., and Norman A. W. (1970). *J. Biol. Chem.* **245**, 4432.

Agus, Z. S., Puschett, J. B., Senesky, D., and Goldberg, M. (1971). *J. Clin Invest.* **50**, 617.

Albright, F. (1947). *Recent Progr. Horm. Res.* **1**, 293.

Albright, F., and Elsworth R. J. (1929) *J. Clin Invest.* **7**, 183.

Albright, F., and Reifenstein, E. C. (1948). "The Parathyroid Glands and Metabolic Bone Disease." Williams & Wilkins, Baltimore, Maryland. (1968).

Albright, F., Bauer, W., and Aub, J. C. (1931). *J. Clin. Invest.* **10**, 187.

Albright, F., Bloomberg, E., and Smith, P. H. (1940). *Trans. Ass. Amer. Physicians* **55**, 298.

Alcock, N. W., and Reid, J. A. (1969). *Biochem. J.* **112**, 511.

Alcock, N. W., and Shils, M. E. (1969). *Biochem. J.* **112**, 505.

Aldred, J. P., Kleszynski, K. R., and Bastian, J. W. (1970). *Proc. Soc. Exp. Biol. Med.* **134**, 1175.

Aliapoulios, M. A., Goldhaber, P., and Munson, P. L. (1966). *Science* **151**, 330.

Altman, P. A., and Dittmer, D. S., Eds. (1968). "Metabolism." *Fed. Amer. Soc. Exp. Biol.*, Bethesda, Maryland.

Anderson, A. P., and Oastler, E. G. (1938). *J. Physiol. (London)* **92**, 124.

Anderson, C. E., and Parker, J. (1966). *J. Bone Joint Surg., Amer. Vol.* **48**, 899.

Anderson, H. C. (1969). *J. Cell Biol.* **41**, 59.

Anderson, H. C., Matsuzawa, T., Sajdera, S. W., and Ali, S.Y. (1970). *Trans. N.Y. Acad. Sci.* [2] **32**, 619.

Antoniori, L. D., Eisner, G. M., Slotkoff, L. M., and Lilienfeld, L. S. (1969). *J. Lab. Clin. Med.* **74**, 410.

Antoniori, L. D., Shalhoub, R. J., Gallagher, P., and O'Connell, J. M. B. (1971). *Amer. J. Physiol.* **220**, 816.

Applebaum, E. (1943). *J. Dent. Res.* **22**, 7.

Ardaillou, R., Fillastre, J. T., Milhaud, G., Ronsselet, F., Delaunay, F., and Richet, G. (1969). *Proc. Soc. Exp. Biol. Med.* **131**, 56.

Armstrong, W. D. (1945). *J. Dent. Res.* **24**, 192.

Armstrong, W. D., and Singer, L. (1965). *Clin. Orthop. Related Res.* **38**, 179.

Armstrong, W. D., Johnson, J. A., Singer, L., Lienke, R. J., and Premer, M. L. (1952). *Amer. J. Physiol.* **171**, 641.

Arnaud, C., Rasmussen, H., and Anast, C. (1966). *J. Clin. Invest.* **45**, 1955.

Arnold, J. S., Jee, W. S. S., and Johnson, K. (1956). *Amer. J. Anat.* **99**, 291.

Artom, C., Sarzana, G., and Segré, E. (1938). *Arch. Int. Physiol.* **47**, 245.

Asgar, K. (1956). *J. Dent. Res.* **35**, 742.

Atkinson, H. F., and Harcourt, J. K. (1962). *Nature (London)* **195**, 508.

Au, W. Y. W., and Raisz, L. G. (1965). *Amer. J. Physiol.* **209**, 637.

Aubert, J. P., and Bronner, F. (1965). *Biophys. J.* **5**, 349.

Aubert, J. P., Bronner, F., and Richelle, L. J. (1963). *J. Clin. Invest.* **42**, 885.

Aurbach, G. D;, and Chase, L. R. (1970). *Fed. Proc., Fed. Amer. Soc. Exp. Biol.* **29**, 1179.

Averill, H. M., and Bibby, B. G. (1964). *J. Dent. Res.* **43**, 1150.

Avery, J. K., Visser, R. L., and Knapp, D. E. (1961). *J. Dent. Res.* **40**, 1004.

Avioli, L. V., and Prockop, D. J. (1967). *J. Clin. Invest.* **46**, 217.

Avioli, L. V., Williams, T. F., Lund, J., and DeLuca, H. G. (1967). *J. Clin. Invest.* **46**, 1907.

Avioli, L. V., Burge, S. J., Scott, S., and Shieber, W. (1969a). *Amer. J. Physiol.* **216**, 939.

Avioli, L. V., Scott, S., Lee, S. W., and DeLuca, H. F. (1969b). *Science* **166**, 1154.

Bachra, B. N., and Wöstmann, B. S. J. (1955). *Arch. Int. Physiol. Biochim.* **63**, 273.

Bacon, J. A., Patrick, H., and Hansard, S. L. (1956). *Proc. Soc. Exp. Biol. Med.* **93**, 349.

Bader, H. (1964). *Biophysik* **1**, 370.

Bailey, K. (1946) *Nature (London)* **157**, 368.

Bailey, K. (1948). *Biochem. J.* **43**, 271.

Bailey, K., Gutfreund, H., and Ogston, A. G. (1948). *Biochem. J.* **43**, 279.

Bailie, J. M;, and Irving, J. T. (1955). *Acta Med. Scand.* **152**, Suppl. 306, 1.

Baker, P. F., Blaustein, M. P., Hodgkin, A. L., and Steinhardt, R. A. (1969). *J. Physiol (London)* **200**, 431.

Baker, P. F., Hodgkin, A. L., and Ridgway, E. B. (1971). *J. Physiol (London)* **218**, 709.

Baker, P. T., and Mazess, R. B. (1963). *Science* **142**, 1466.

Banerjee, S., and Ghosh, P. K. (1961). *Proc. Soc. Exp. Biol. Med.* **107**, 275.

Banks, P. (1967). *J. Physiol. (London)* **193**, 631.

Banks, P., Biggins, R., Bishop, R., Christian, B., and Currie, N. (1969). *J. Physiol. (London)* **200**, 797.

Barclay, J. A., Cooke, W. T., and Kenney, K. S. (1947). *Acta Med. Scand.* **128**, 500.

Barnicot, N. A. (1948). *J. Anat.* **82**, 233.

Barnicot, N. A. (1950). *J. Anat.* **84**, 374.

Barnicot, N. A. (1951). *J. Anat.* **85**, 120.

Barnum, C. P., and Armstrong, W. D. (1941). *J. Dent. Res.* **20**, 232.

Barreras, R. F., and Donaldson, R. M. (1967). *Gastroenterology* **52**, 670.

Baskin, R. J. (1971). *J. Cell Biol.* **48**, 49.

Bates, W. K., Awapara, J., and Talmage, R. V. (1964). *Proc. Soc. Exp. Biol. Med.* **115**, 650.

Bauer, W., Aub, J. C., and Albright, F. (1929). *J. Exp. Med.* **49**, 145.

Bauer, W., Albright, F., and Aub, J. C. (1930). *J. Clin. Invest.* **8**, 229.

Bavetta, L. A., and Bernick, S. (1955). *J. Amer. Dent. Ass.* **50**, 427.

Bavetta, L. A., and Bernick, S. (1956). *Oral Surg., Oral Med. Oral Pathol.* **9**, 308.

Bavetta, L. A., Bernick, S., Geiger, E., and Bergen, W. (1954). *J. Dent. Res.* **33**, 309.

Bawden, J. W., and McIver, F. T. (1964). *J. Dent. Res.* **43**, 563.

Baylink, D. J., and Bernstein, D; S. (1967). *Clin. Orthop. Related Res.* **55**, 51.

Baylor, C. H., Van Alstine, H. E., Kentman, E. H., and Bassett, S. H. (1950). *J. Clin. Invest.* **29**, 1167.

Beal, V. A. (1954). *J. Nutr.* **53**, 499.

Beck, N. P., DeRubertis, F., Michelis, M. F., Fusco, R. D., Field, J. B., and Davis, B. B. (1970). *J. Lab. Clin. Med.* **76**, 1005.

Becks, H., and Ryder, W. B. (1931). *Arch. Pathol.* **12**, 358.

Becks, H., Simpson, M. E., and Evans, H. M. (1945). *Anat. Rec.* **92**, 121.

Becks, H., Collins, D. A., Simpson, M. E., and Evans, H. M. (1946). *Arch. Pathol.* **41**, 457.

Becks, H., Scow, R. O., Simpson, M. E., Asling, C. W., Li, C. H., and Evans, H. M. (1950). *Anat. Rec.* **107**, 299.

Begum, A., and Pereira, S. M. (1969). *Brit. J. Nutr.* **23**, 905.

Bélanger, L. F., and Migicovsky, B. B. (1960). *Develop. Biol.* **2**, 329.

Bélanger, L. F., and Migicovsky, B. B. (1963). *J. Histochem. Cytochem.* **11**, 734.

Bélanger, L. F., and Robichon, J. (1964). *J. Bone Joint Surg., Amer. Vol.* **46**, 1008.

Bélanger, L. F., Semba, T., Tolnai, S., Copp, D. H., Krook, L., and Gries, C. (1966). *Calcif. Tissues 1965., Proc. Eur. Symp., 3rd, 1965* p. 1.

Bell, N. H., and Stern, P. H. (1970). *Amer. J. Physiol.* **218**, 64.

Bell, N. H., Barrett, R. J., and Patterson, R. (1966). *Proc. Soc. Exp. Biol. Med.* **123**, 114.

Bendall, J. R. (1952). *Nature (London)* **170**, 1058.

Bendall, J. R. (1953). *J. Physiol. (London)* **121**, 232.

Benowitz, N. L., and Terepka, A. R. (1968). *Proc. Soc. Exp. Biol. Med.* **129**, 46.

Berg, G. G. (1964). *J. Histochem. Cytochem.* **12**, 341.

Bergeim, O. (1926). *J. Biol. Chem.* **70**, 51.

Berman, M. E., Shahn, E., and Weiss, M. F. (1962). *Biophys. J.* **2**, 275.

Bernard, G. W., and Pease, D. C. (1969). *Amer. J. Anat.* **125**, 271.

Bernstein, D., Kleeman, C. R., and Maxwell, M. H. (1963). *Proc. Soc. Exp. Biol. Med.* **112**, 353.

Bernstein, D. S., and Handler, P. (1958). *Proc. Soc. Exp. Biol. Med.* **99**, 339.

Bertaud, W. S;, Rayns, D. G;, and Simpson, F. O. (1970). *J. Cell Sci.* **6**, 537.

Bessey, O. A., King, C. J., Quinn, E. J., and Sherman, H. C. (1935). *J. Biol. Chem.* **111**, 115.

Better, O. S., Gonick, H. C., Chapman, L. C., Varrady, P. D., and Kleeman, C. R. (1966). *Proc. Soc. Exp. Biol. Med.* **121**, 592.

Bevelander, G., and Nakahara, H. (1966). *Anat. Rec.* **156**, 303.

Bhandarkar, S. D., Bluhm, M., MacGregor, J., and Nordin, B. E. C. (1961). *Brit. Med. J.* **2**, 1639.

Birge, S. J., Keutmann, H. T., Cautrecasas, P., and Whedon, G. D. (1967). *N. Engl. J. Med.* **276**, 445.

Birks, R. I., and Cohen, M. W. (1968a). *Proc. Roy. Soc. Ser. B* **170**, 381.

Birks, R. I., and Cohen, M. W. (1968b). *Proc. Roy. Soc., Ser. B* **170**, 401.

Blau, M., Spencer, H., Swernov, J., Greenberg, J., and Laszlo, D. (1957), *J. Nutr.* **61**, 507.

Blaustein, M. P., and Hodgkin, A. L. (1969). *J. Physiol* (*London*) **200**, 497.

Blioch, Z. L., Glagoleva, I. M. Liberman, E. A., and Nenasher, V. A. (1968). *J. Physiol.* (*London*) **199**, 11.

Bloom, M. A., Domm, L. V., Nabandov, A. V., and Bloom, W. (1958). Amer. J. Anat. **102**, 411.

Bloomquist, E., and Curtis, B. A. (1972). *J. Gen. Physiol.* **59**, 476.

Blunt, J. W., and DeLuca, H. F. (1969). *Biochemistry* **8**, 671.

Blunt, J. W., DeLuca, H. F., and Schnoes, H. K. (1968). *Biochemistry* **7**, 3317.

Blythe, W. B., Gitelman, H. J., and Welt, L. G. (1968). *Amer. J. Physiol.* **214**, 52.

Bocciarelli, D. S. (1970). *Calif. Tissues Res.* **5**, 261.

Bodansky, M;, and Duff, V. B. (1941). *J. Nutr.* **22**, 25.

Boelter, M. D. D., and Greenberg, D. M. (1941). *J. Nutr.* **21**, 61.

Bohatirchuk, F. (1966). *Amer. J. Med.* **41**, 836.

Bonucci, E. (1967). *J. Ultrastruct. Res.* **20**, 33.

Bonucci, E. (1969). *Calif. Tissues Res.* **3**, 38.

Bonucci, E. (1970). *Z. Zellforsch. Mikrosk, Anat.* **103**, 192.

Borle, A. B. (1968). *J. Cell Biol.* **36**, 567.

Borle, A. B., Nichols, B., and Nichols, G. (1960). *J. Biol. Chem.* **235**, 1211.

Borle, A. B., Keutmann, H. T., and Neuman, W. F. (1963). *Amer. J. Physiol.* **204**, 705.

Borowitz, J. L. (1969). *Biochem. Pharmacol.* **18**, 715.

Boyle, I. T., Gray, R. W., and DeLuca, H. F. (1971). *Proc. Nat. Acad. Sci. U.S.* **68**, 2131.

Bozler, E. (1954). *J. Gen. Physiol.* **38**, 149.

Bradbury, M. W. B., Kleeman, C. R., Bagdoyan, H., and Berberlain, A. (1968). *J. Lab. Clin. Med.* **71**, 884.

Bradham, L., Holt, A. D., and Sims, M., (1970). *Biochim. Biophys. Acta* **201**, 250.

Braham, J. E., Tijada, C., Guzmán, M. A., and Bressani, R. (1961). *J. Nutr.* **74**, 363.

Bredderman, P. J. (1971). Thesis, Cornell University, Ithaca, New York.

Breen, M., and Freeman, S. (1961). *Amer. J. Physiol.* **200**, 341.

Breiter, H., Mills, R., Dwight, J., McKey, B., Armstrong, W., and Outhouse, J. (1941). *J. Nutr.* **21**, 351.

Breiter, H., Mills, R., Rutherford, E., Armstrong, W., and Outhouse, J. (1942). *J. Nutr.* **23**, 1.

Brewer, H. B., Keutmann, H. T., Potts, J. T., Reisfeld, R. A., Schlueter, R., and Munson, P. L. (1968). *J. Biol. Chem.* **243**, 5739.

Brewer, H. B., Schlueter, R. J., and Aldred, J. P. (1970). *J. Biol. Chem.* **245**, 4232.

Bricker, M. L., Smith, M. J., Hamilton, T. S;, and Mitchell, H. H. (1949). *J. Nutr.* **39**, 445.

Brierley, G. P., Murer, E., and Bachmann, E. (1964). *Arch. Biochem. Biophys.* **105**, 82.

Brine, C. L., and Johnston, F. A. (1955). *Amer. J. Clin. Nutr.* **3**, 418.

Brinkman, A. S., Massry, S. G., and Coburn, J. W. (1971). *Amer. J. Physiol.* **220**, 44.

Bronner, F. (1957). *Fed. Proc., Fed. Amer. Soc. Exp. Biol.* **16**, 158.

Bronner, F. (1960). *Science* **132**, 472.

Bronner, F. (1964). *In* "Mineral Metabolism" (C. L. Comar and F. Bronner, eds.), Vol. 2A, p. 341. Academic Press, New York.

Bronner, F. (1967). *Trans. N.Y. Acad. Sci.* [2] **29**, 502.

Bronner, F. (1973). *In* "Engineering Principles in Physiology" (J. H. U. Brown and D. Gann, eds.), Vol. I, pp. 227–248. Academic Press, New York.

Bronner, F., and Aubert, J. P. (1965). *Amer. J. Physiol.* **209**, 887.

Bronner, F., and Lemaire, R. (1969). *Calcif. Tissue Res.* **3**, 238.

Bronner, F., and Thompson, D. D. (1961). *J. Physiol (London)* **157**, 232.

Bronner, F., Harris, R. F., Maletskos, C. J., and Benda, C. E. (1956). *J. Nutr.* **59**, 393.

Bronner, F., Sammon, P. J., Stacey, R. E., and Shah, B. G. (1967). *Biochem. Med.* **1**, 261.

Bronner, F., Sammon P. J., Nichols, C., Stacey, R. E., and Shah, B. G. (1968). *In* "Parathyroid Hormone and Thyrocalcitonin (Calcitonin)" (R. V. Talmage and L. R. Bélanger, eds.), p. 353. Excerpta Med. Found., Amsterdam.

Brown, D. M., Perey, D. Y., Dent, P. B., and Good, R. A. (1969). *Proc. Soc. Exp. Biol. Med.* **130**, 1001.

Brown, E. B., and Prasad, A. S. (1957). *Amer. J. Physiol.* **190**, 462.

Brown, H. (1926). *J. Biol. Chem.* **68**, 729.

Brown, W. E., Smith, J. P., Lehr, J. R., and Frazier, A. W. (1962). *Nature (London)* **196**, 1050.

Buchanan, G. D., Kraintz, F. W., and Talmage, R. V. (1959). *Proc. Soc. Exp. Biol. Med.* **101**, 306.

Buckle, R. M. (1969). *J. Physiol. (London)* **202**, 33P (Abstract in program).

Bullamore, J. R., Wilkinson, R., Gallagher, J. C., Nordin, B. E. C., and Marshall, D. H. (1970). *Lancet* **2**, 535.

Bunge, G. (1898). "Lehrbuch der physiologischen Chemie," 4th ed., p. 118. Leipzig.

Bürger, M., and Schlomka, G. (1939). Quoted *in* "Problems of Aging, Biological and Medical Aspects" (by E. V. Cowdry), p. 612. Baillière, London.

Burke, B. S., Reed, R. B., VanDen Burg, A. S., and Stuart, H. C. (1962), *Amer. J. Clin. Nutr.* **10**, 79.

Burnette, J. C., Simpson, D. M., Chandler, D. C., and Bawden, J. W. (1968). *J. Dent. Res.* **47**, 444.

Burns, C. M. (1933). *Biochem. J.* **27**, 22.

Burstone, M. S. (1960). *In* "Calcification in Biological Systems," Publ. No. 64, pp. 217–243. Amer. Ass. Advan. Sci., Washington, D.C.

Bussolati, G., and Pearse, A. G. E. (1967). *J. Endocrinol.* **37**, 205.

Byfield, P. G. H., Turner, K., Galante, L., Gudmundsson, T. V., MacIntyre, I., Riniker, B., Neher, R., Maier, R., and Kahnt, F. W. (1969). *Biochem. J.* **111**, 13P.

Cameron, D. A. (1961). *J. Bone Joint Surg., Brit. Vol.* **43**, 590.

Cameron, D. A. (1963). *Clin. Orthop. Related Res.* **26**, 199.

Campbell, H. L., Bessey, O. A., and Sherman, H. C. (1935). *J. Biol. Chem.* **110**, 703.

Campbell, J. R., and Douglas, T. A. (1965). *Brit. J. Nutr.* **19**, 339.

Campo, R. D., Tourtelotte, C. D., and Bielen, R. J. (1969). *Biochim. Biophys. Acta* **177**, 501.

Canas, F., Brand, J. S., Neuman, W. F;, and Terepka, A. R. (1969). *Amer. J. Physiol.* **216**, 1092.

Capen, C. C., and Young, D. M. (1969). *Amer. J. Pathol.* **57**, 365.

Carafoli, E., and Lehninger, A. L. (1971). *Biochem. J.* **122**, 681.

Care, A. D. (1968). *Fed. Proc., Fed. Amer. Soc. Exp. Biol.* **27**, 153.

Care, A. D., Sherwood, L. M., Potts, J. T., and Aurbach, G. D. (1966). *Nature (London)* **209**, 55.

Care, A. D., Copper, C. W., Duncan, T., and Orimo, H. (1968). *In* "Parathyroid Hormone and Thyrocalcitonin (Calcitonin)" (R. V. Talmage and L. F. Bélanger, eds.), p. 417. Excerpta Med. Found., Amsterdam.

Carlsson, A. (1951). *Acta Pharmacol. Toxicol.* **7**, Suppl 1, p. 1.

Carlström, D., and Glas, J. E. (159). Biochim. Biophys. Acta **35**, 46.

Carneiro, J., and Leblond, C. P. (1959). *Exp. Cell Res.* **18**, 291.

Carr, C. W. (1953). *Arch. Biochem. Biophys.* **43**, 147.

Carrasquer, G., and Brodsky, W. A. (1961). *Amer. J. Physiol.* **201**, 499.

Cartier, P., and Lanzetta, A. (1961). *Bull. Soc. Chim. Biol.* **43**, 981.

Carvalho, A. P. (1966). *J. Cell. Physiol.* **67**, 73.

Carvalho, A. P. (1968a). *J. Gen Physiol.* **51**, 427.

Carvalho, A. P. (1968b). *J. Gen. Physiol.* **52**, 622.

Chance, B. (1965). *J. Biol Chem.* **240**, 2729.

Chance, B., and Azzi, A. (1969). *Ann. N.Y. Acad. Sci.* **147**, 805.

Chang, H-Y. (1951). *Anat. Rec.* **111**, 23.

Chappell, J. B., and Crofts, A. R. (1965). *Biochem. J.* **95**, 378.

Chattopadhyay, H., and Freeman, S. (1965). *Amer. J. Physiol.* **208**, 1036.

Chayen, J., Chayen, R;, Cunningham, G. J., and Bitensky, L. (1961). *Pathol. Biol.* **9**, 925.

Cheeseman, E. M., Copping, A. M., and Prebble, P. M. (1964). *Brit. J. Nutr.* **18**, 147.

Chen, P. S., and Bosmann, H. B. (1955). *J. Nutr.* **87**, 148.

Chen, P. S., and Neuman, W. F. (1955). *Amer. J. Physiol.* **180**, 623 and 632.

Chen, T. C., Weber, J. C., and DeLuca, H. F. (1970). *J. Biol. Chem.* **245**, 3776.

Chutkow, J. G. (1968). *Proc. Soc. Exp. Biol. Med.* **128**, 555.

Claasen, V., and Wöstman, B. S. (1953). *Biochim. Biophys. Acta* **12**, 557.

Clark, I., and Geoffroy, R. (1958). *J. Biol. Chem.* **233**, 203.

Clark, I., and Smith, M. R. (1964). *J. Biol. Chem.* **239**, 1266.

Clark, J. D., Zatzman, M. L., and Kenny, A. D. (1968). *Biochem. J.* **108**, 25P.

Clegg, R. E., and Hein, R. E. (1953). *Poultry Sci.* **32**, 867.

Coates, M. E., and Holdsworth, E. S. (1961). *Brit. J. Nutr.* **15**, 131.

Cohn, D. V., and Forscher, B. K. (1961). *Biochim. Biophys. Acta* **52**, 596.

Cohn, D. V., and Forscher, B. K. (1962). *Biochim. Biophys. Acta* **65**, 20.

Cohn, D. V., Bawden, R. and Eller, G. (1967). *J. Biol. Chem.* **242**, 1253.

Cohn, S. H., Bozzo, S. R., Jesseph, J. E., Constantinides, C., Huene, D. R., and Gusmano, E. A. (1965). *Radiat. Res.* **26**, 319.

Cohn, S. H., Danbrowski, C. S., Hauser, W., and Atkins, H. L. (1968). *Amer. J. Clin. Nutr.* **21**, 1246.

Collip, J. B. (1926). *Medicine (Baltimore)* **5**, 1.

Colomo, F., Rahamimoff, R. (1968). *J. Physiol. (London)* **198**, 203.

Consolazio, C. F., Matoush, L. O., Nelson, R. A., Hackler, L. R., and Preston, E. E. (1962). *J. Nutr.* **78**, 78.

Constantin, L. L., and Podolsky, R. J. (1966). *Nature (London)* **210**, 483.

Constantin, L. L., Franzini-Armstrong, C., and Podolsky, R. J. (1965). *Science* **147**, 158.

Coons, C. M. (1935). *Okla., Agr. Exp. Sta., Bull.* **223**, 113.

Coons, C. M., and Coons, R. R. (1935). *J. Nutr.* **10**, 289.

Cooper, W. E. G. (1968). *Arch. Oral biol.* **13**, 27.

Copp, D. H. (1957). *Amer. J. Med.* **22**, 275.

Copp, D. H. (1960). *In* "Bone as a Tissue" (K. Rodahl, J. T. Nicholson, and E. M. Brown, eds.), p. 289. McGraw-Hill, New York.

Copp, D. H. (1969). *In* "Mineral Metabolism" (C. L. Comar and F. Bronner, eds.), Vol. 3, p. 453. Academic Press, New York.

Copp, D. H. (1970). *Annu. Rev. Physiol.* **32**, 61.

Copp, D. H., and Cameron, E. C. (1962). *Science* **134**, 2038.

Copp, D. H., and Cheyney, B. (1962). *Nature (London)* **193**, 381.

Copp, D. H., and Davidson, A. G. F. (1961). *Proc. Soc. Exp. Biol. Med.* **107**, 342.

Copp, D. H., and Kuczerpa, A. V. (1968). *In* "Les Tissus Calcifiés. Fifth European Symposium" (G. Milhaud, M. Owen, and H. J. J. Blackwood, eds.), p. 167. Soc. d'Édition d'Enseignment Supérieur, Paris.

Copp, D. H., Kuczerpa, A., and Bélanger, L. (1965). *Proc. Can. Fed. Biol. Soc.* **4**, 17.

Copp, D. H., Cockcroft, D. W., and Kuch, Y. (1967). *Science* **158**, 924.

Corradino, R. A., and Wasserman, R. H. (1968a). *Arch. Biochem. Biophys.* **125**, 378.

Corradino, R. A., and Wasserman, R. H. (1968b). *Arch. Biochem. Biophys.* **126**, 957.

Corradino, R. A., and Wasserman, R. H. (1970a). *Fed. Proc., Fed. Amer. Soc. Exp. Biol.* **29**, Abst, No. 692, p. 368.

Corradino, R. A., and Wasserman, R. H. (1970b). *Proc. Soc. Exp. Biol. Med.* **133**, 960.

Correll, J. T., and Hughes, J. S. (1933). *J. Biol. Chem.* **103**, 511.

Cotmore, J. M., Nichols, G., and Wuthier, R. E. (1971). *Science* **172**, 1339.

Cotton, W. R., and Hefferren, S. M. (1966). *Arch. Oral Biol.* **11**, 1027.

Cousins, R. J., DeLuca, H. F., and Gray, R. W. (1970). *Biochemistry* **9**, 3649.

Coward, K. H. (1938). "The Biological Standardization of the Vitamins." Ballière, London.

Cox, W. M., and Imboden, M. (1936). *J. Nutr.* **11**, 177.

Craig, J. M. (1959). *AMA Arch. Pathol.* **68**, 306.

Cramer, C. F. (1959). *Proc. Soc. Exp. Biol. Med.* **100**, 364.

Cramer, J. W., and Steenbock, H. (1956). *Arch. Biochem. Biophys.* **63**, 9.

Crawford, J. D., Gribetz, D., and Talbot, N. B. (1955). *Amer. J. Physiol.* **180**, 156.

Crawford, M. D., Gardner, M. J., and Morris, J. N. (1968). *Lancet* **1**, 827.

Crenshaw, M. A., and Heeley, J. D. (1967). *45th Gen. Meet., Int. Ass. Dent. Res.* Abstract No. 119, 65.

Cruess, R. L., and Clark, I. (1965). *Biochem. J.* **96**, 262.

Cruess, R. L., and Clark, I. (1967). *Proc. Soc. Exp. Biol. Med.* **126**, 8.

Curry, D. L., Bennett, L. L., and Grodsky, G. M. (1968). *Amer. J. Physiol.* **214**, 174.

Cushny, A. R. (1917). "The Secretion of Urine." Longmans, London.

Dallas, I., and Nordin, B. E. C. (1962). *Amer. J. Clin. Nutr.* **11**, 263.

Dallemagne, M. J., Bodson, P., and Fabry, C. (1955). *Biochim. Biophys. Acta* **18**, 394.

Dancker, P. (1970). *Pfluegers Arch. gesamte Physiol. Menschen Tiere* **315**, 198.

Danielli, J. F., Fell, H. B., and Kodicek, E. (1945). *Brit. J. Exp. Pathol.* **26**, 367.

Davidson, H. R. (1930). *J. Agri. Sci.* **20**, 233.

Davies, J. S., Widdowson, E. M., and McCance, R. A. (1964). *Brit. J. Nutr.* **18**, 385.

Dawson, J., Weidmann, S. M., and Jones, H. G. (1967). *Biochem. J.* **66**, 116.

Deakins, M. (1942). *J. Dent. Res.* **21**, 429.

Deakins, M., and Burt, R. L. (1944). *J. Biol. Chem.* **156**, 77.

DeAngelis, V. (1969). *Amer. J. Anat.* **124**, 379.

Decker, J. D. (1966). *Amer. J. Anat.* **118**, 591.

deJong, W. F. (1926). *Rec. Trav. Chim. Pays-Bas* **45**, 445.

Delf, E. M., and Tozer, F. M. (1918). *Biochem. J.* **12**, 416.

DeLuca, H. F., and Engstrom, G. W. (1961). *Proc. Nat. Acad. Sci. U.S.* **47**, 1744.

DeLuca, H. F., and Steenbock, H. (1957). *Science* **126**, 258.

DeLuca, H. F., Guroff, G., Steenbock, H., Reiser, S., and Mannatt, M. R. (1961). *J. Nutr.* **75**, 175.

DeLuca, H. F., Weller, M., Blunt, J. W., and Neville, P. F. (1968). *Arch. Biochem. Biophys.* **124**, 122.

Demartini, F. E., Briscoe, A. M., and Ragan, C. (1967). *Proc. Soc. Exp. Biol. Med.* **124**, 320.

deRobertis, E. D. P., and Bennet, A. S. (1954). *Fed. Proc., Fed. Amer. Soc. Exp. Biol.* **13**, 35.

Dessauer, H. C., Fox, W., and Gilbert, N. L. (1956). *Proc. Soc. Exp. Biol. Med.* **92**, 299.

Diamant, B. (1967). *Acta Pharmacol. Toxicol.* **25**, Suppl. 4, 33.

Diamant, B., and Kruger, P. G. (1967). *Acta Physiol. Scand.* **71**, 291.

Diamond, M., and Weinmann, J. P. (1940). "The Enamel of Human Teeth." Columbia Univ. Press, New York.

Dicker, S. E. (1966). *J. Physiol. (London)* **185**, 429.

Dirksen, T. R. (1963). *J. Dent. Res.* **42**, 128.

Dirksen, T. R., and Ikels, K. G. (1964). *J. Dent. Res.* **43**, 246.

DiSalvo, J., and Schubert, M. (1967). *J. Biol. Chem.* **242**, 705.

Dixit, P. K. (1967) *Proc. Soc. Exp. Biol. Med.* **125**, 968.

Dixit, P. K. (1969). *J. Histochem. Cytochem.* **17**, 411.

Dixon, H. H., Davenport, H. A., and Ranson, S. W. (1929). *J. Biol. Chem.* **83**, 739.

Dodds, G. S., and Cameron, H. C. (1934). *Amer. J. Anat.* **55**, 135.

Dodge, F. A., Miledi, R., and Rahamimoff, R. (1969). *J. Physiol, (London)* **200**, 267.

Dols, M. J. L., Jansen, B. C. P., Sizoo, G. J., and DeVries, J. (1937). *Proc. Kon. Ned. Akad. Wetensch.* **40**, 547.

Donelson, E., Nims, B., Hunscher, H. A., and Macy, I. G. (1931). *J. Biol. Chem.* **91**, 675.

Douglas, W. W. (1963). *Nature (London)* **197**, 81.

Douglas, W. W. (1968). *Brit. J. Pharmacol.* **34**, 451.

Douglas, W. W., and Poisner, A. M. (1962). *J. Physiol. (London)* **162**, 385.

Douglas, W. W., and Poisner, A. M. (1963). *J. Physiol. (London)* **165**, 528.

Douglas, W. W., and Poisner, A. M. (1964a). *J. Physiol. (London)* **172**, 1.

Douglas, W. W., and Poisner, A. M. (1964b). *J. Physiol. (London)* **172**, 19.

Douglas, W. W., and Rubin, R. P. (1961). *J. Physiol. (London)* **159**, 40.

Douglas, W. W., and Rubin, R. P. (1963). *J. Physiol. (London)* **167**, 288.

Douglas, W. W., and Rubin, R. P. (1964). *J. Physiol. (London)* **175**, 231.

Douša, T., and Rychlík, I. (1968). *Biochim. Biophys. Acta* **158**, 484.

Dowdle, E. B., Schachter, D., and Schenker, H. (1960). *Amer. J. Physiol.* **198**, 269.

Drahota, Z., Carafoli, E., Rossi, C. S., Gamble, R. L., and Lehninger, A. L. (1965). *J. Biol. Chem.* **240**, 2712.

Dreisbach, R. H. (1964). *Amer. J. Physiol.* **207**, 1015.

Drescher, D., DeLuca, H. F., and Imrie, M. H. (1969). *Arch. Biochem. Biophys.* **130**, 657.

Drummond, K. N., and Michael, A. F. (1964). *Nature (London)* **201**, 1333.

Duarte, C. G., and Watson, J. F. (1967). *Amer. J. Physiol.* **212**, 1355.

Dudley, H. R., and Spiro, D. (1961). *J. Biophys. Biochem. Cytol.* **11**, 627.

Durkin, J. F., Irving, J. T., and Heeley, J. D. (1971). *Arch. Oral Biol.* **16**, 827.

Dymsza, H. A., Reussner, G., and Thiessen, R. (1959). *J. Nutr.* **69**, 419.

Eanes, E. D. (1970). *Calcif. Tissue. Res.* **5**, 133.

Eanes, E. D., and Posner, A. S. (1968). *Calcif. Tissue Res.* **2**, 38.

Eanes, E. D., Gillessen, I. H., and Posner, A. S. (1965). *Nature (London)* **208**, 365.

Eastoe, J. E. (1956). *In* "The Biochemistry and Physiology of Bone" (G. H. Bourne, ed.), pp. 81–105. Academic Press, New York.

Eastoe, J. E. (1963). *Arch. Oral Biol.* **8**, 633.

Ebashi, S. (1960). *J. Biochem. (Tokyo)* **48**, 150.

Ebashi, S. (1961a). *Tokyo J. Med. Sci.* **69**, 65.

Ebashi, S. (1961b). *J. Biochem. (Tokyo)* **50**, 236.

Ebashi, S. (1961c). *Progr. Theor. Phys., Suppl.* **17**, 35.

Ebashi, S., and Ebashi, F. (1964). *J. Biochem. (Tokyo)* **55**, 604.

Ebashi, S., and Endo, M. (1968). *Progr. Biophys. Mol. Biol.* **18**, 125.

Ebashi, S., and Kodama, A. (1965). *J. Biochem. (Tokyo)* **58**, 107.

Ebashi, S., and Kodama, A. (1966). *J. Biochem. (Tokyo)* **59**, 425.

Ebashi, S., and Lipmann, F. (1962). *J. Cell. Biol.* **14**, 389.

Ebashi, S., Ebashi, F., and Kodama, A. (1967). *J. Biochem. (Tokyo)* **62**, 137.

Economou-Mavrou, C., and McCance, R. A. (1958). *Biochem. J.* **68**, 573.

Eeg-Larsen, N. (1956). *Acta Physiol. Scand.* **38**, Suppl. 128.

Eisenberg, E. (1965). *J. Clin. Invest.* **44**, 942.

Eisenmann, D. R., and Yaeger, J. A. (1972). *Arch. Oral Biol.* **17**, 987.

Eisenstein, R., and Passavoy, M. (1964). *Proc. Soc. Exp. Biol. Med.* **117**, 77.

Ellsworth, R., and Howard, J. E. (1934). *Bull. Johns Hopkins Hosp.* **55**, 296.

El-Maraghi, N. R. H., Platt, B. S., and Stewart, R. J. C. (1965). *Brit. J. Nutr.* **19**, 491.

Endo, M. (1964). *Nature (London)* **202**, 1115.

Engfeldt, B., and Essler-Hammarlund, E. (1956). *Acta Odontol. Scand.* **14**, 273.

Engstrom, G. W., and DeLuca, H. F. (1964). *Biochemistry* **3**, 379.

Enlow, D. H., and Conklin, J. L. (1964). *Anat. Rec.* **148**, 279.

Enlow, D. H., Conklin, J. L., and Bang, S. (1965). *Clin. Orthop. Related Res.* **38**, 157.

Erdheim, J. (1906). *Mitt. Grenzgeb. Med. Chir.* **16**, 632.

Ericson, A. T., Clegg, R. E., and Hein, R. E. (1955). *Science* **122**, 199.

Ettori, J., and Scoggan, S. M. (1959). *Nature (London)* **184**, 1315.

Evans, H. M., Becks, H., Asling, C. W., Simpson, M. E., and Li, C. H. (1948). *Growth* **12**, 43.

Exton-Smith, A. N., Hodkinson, H. M., and Stanton, B. R. (1966). *Lancet* **2**, 999.

Fairbanks, B. W., and Mitchell, H. H. (1936). *J. Nutr.* **11**, 551.

Fairney, A., and Weir, A. A. (1970). *J. Endocrinol.* **48**, 337.

Falk, G., and Fatt, P. (1964). *Proc. Roy. Soc. Ser. B* **160**, 69.

Farese, R. V. (1971). *Science* **173**, 447.

Fatt, P., and Katz, B. (1952). *J. Physiol. (London)* **117**, 109.

Fearnhead, R. W. (1960). *J. Dent. Res.* **39**, 1104.

Fearnhead, R. W. (1963). *Arch. Oral Biol.* **8**, suppl, p. 257.

Feaster, J. P., Hansard, S. L., Outler, J. C., and Davis, G. K. (1956). *J. Nutr.* **58**, 399.

Fehling, H. (1877). *Arch. Gynaekol.* **11**, 523.

Fell. H. B., and Mellanby, E. (1952). *J. Physiol. (London)* **116**, 320.

Ferguson, H. W., and Hartles, R. L. (1964). *Arch. Oral Biol.* **9**, 447.

Ferguson, R. K., and Wolbach, R. A. (1967). *Amer. J. Physiol.* **212**, 1123.

Fernández-Morán, H., and Engström, A. (1957). *Biochim. Biophys. Acta* **23**, 260.

Filer, L. J., and Foman, S. J. (1966). *Proc. 7th. Int. Congr. Nutr.*, 62.

Finkelstein, J. D., and Schachter, D. (1962). *Amer. J. Physiol.* **203**, 873.

Finn, S. B., and Jamison, H. C. (1967). *J. Amer. Dent. Ass.* **74**, 987.

Firschein, H. E. (1970). *Amer. J. Physiol.* **219**, 1183.

Fischman, D. A., and Hay, E. D. (1962). *Anat. Rec.* **143**, 329.

Fish, E. W., and Harris, L. J. (1934). *Phil. Trans. Roy. Soc. London, Ser. B* **223**, 489.

Fitton-Jackson, S., and Randall, J. T. (1956). *Nature (London)* **178**, 798.

Flanagan, B., and Nichols, G. (1969). *J. Clin. Invest.* **48**, 595.

Fleisch, H. (1964). *Clin. Orthop. Related Res.* **32**, 170.

Fleisch, H., and Bisaz, S. (1962a). *Amer. J. Physiol.* **203**, 671.

Fleisch, H., and Bisaz, S. (1962b). *Helv. Physiol. Pharmacol. Acta* **20**, 52.

Fleisch, H., and Neuman, W. F. (1961). *Amer. J. Physiol.* **200**, 1296.

Fleisch, H., Straumann, F., Schenk, R., Bisaz, S., and Allgower, M. (1966). *Amer. J. Physiol.* **211**, 821.

Fleisch, H., Russell, R. G. G., Bisaz, S., Termine, J. D., and Posner, A. S. (1968). *Calcif. Tissue Res.* **2**, 49.

Flores, M., and Garcia, B. (1960). *Brit. J. Nutr.* **14**, 207.

Follis, R. H. (1943). *Arch. Pathol.* **35**, 579.

Follis, R. H. (1951). *Proc. Soc. Exp. Biol. Med.* **76**, 722; **78**, 723.

Food and Agriculture Organization. (1962). *World Health Organ. Tech. Rep. Ser.* **230**.

Food and Nutrition Board. (1964). *Nat. Acad. Sci.—Nat. Res. Coun. Publ.* **1146**

Forbes, E. B., Schulz, J. A., Hunt, C. A., Winter, A. R., and Remler, R. F. (1922). *J. Biol. Chem.* **52**, 281.

Forbes, R. M. (1963). *J. Nutr.* **80**, 321.

Forbes, R. M., Cooper, A. R., and Mitchell, H. H. (1953), *J. Biol. Chem.* **203**, 359.

Forbes, R. M., Mitchell, H. H., and Cooper, R. (1956). *J. Biol. Chem.* **223**, 969.

Forssmann, W. G., and Girardier, L. (1970). *J. Cell Biol.* **44**, 1.

Foster, G. V., Baghdiantz, A., Kumar, M. A., Slack, E., Soliman, H. A., and MacIntyre, I. (1964). *Nature (London)* **202**, 1303.

Foulks, J. (1956). *Fed. Proc., Fed. Amer. Soc. Exp. Biol.* **15**, 65.

Foulks, J. G., and Perry, F. A. (1959). *Amer. J. Physiol.* **196**, 567.

Fournier, P. (1954). *C. R. Acad. Sci.* **238**, 509.

Francis, M. D., Russell, R. G. G., and Fleisch, H. (1969). *Science* **165**, 1264.

François, P. (1961). *J. Physiol. (Paris)* **53**, 343.

François, C. J., Glimcher, M. J., and Krane, S. M. (1967). *Nature (London)* **214**, 621.

Frandsen, A. M. (1963). *Acta Odontol. Scand.* **21**, 19.

Frandsen, A. M., and Becks, H. (1962). *Oral Surg., Oral Med. Oral Pathol.* **15**, 474.

Frandsen, A. M., Nelson, M. M., Sulon, E., Becks, H., and Evans, H. M. (1954). *Anat. Rec.* **119**, 247.

Frank, R. M. (1961). *Arch. Oral Biol.* **4**, 29.

Frank, R. M., and Sognnaes, R. F. (1960). *Arch. Oral Biol.* **1**, 339.

Frankenhaeuser, B. (1957). *J. Physiol. (London)* **137**, 245.

Frankenhaeuser, B., and Hodgkin, A. L. (1957). *J. Physiol. (London)* **137**, 218.

Franzini-Armstrong, C. (1970). *J. Cell Biol.* **47**, 64A.

Franzini-Armstrong C. (1971). *J. Cell Biol.* **49**, 196.

Franzini-Armstrong, C., and Porter, K. R. (1964). *J. Cell Biol.* **22**, 675.

Fraser, D., Jaco, N. T., Yendt, E. R., Munn, J. D., and Liu, E. (1957). *Amer. J. Dis. Child.* **93**, 84.

Freeman, S., and McLean, F. C. (1941). *Arch. Pathol.* **32**, 387.

Friedman, J., and Raisz, L. G. (1965). *Science* **150**, 1465.

Friend, B. (1967). *Amer. J. Clin. Nutr.* **20**, 907.

Fries, B. A., Ruben, S., Perlman, I., and Chaikoff, I. L. (1938). *J. Biol. Chem.* **123**, 587.

Fuchs, A. R., and Fuchs, F. (1954). *Acta Physiol. Scand.* **30**, 191.

Fujita, K. (1954). *Folia Pharmacol. Jap.* **50**, 183.

Fullmer, C. S., and Wasserman, R. H. (1972). *Fed. Proc. Fed. Amer. Soc. Exp. Biol.* **31**, 693.

Fullmer, H. M. (1964). *J. Histochem. Cytochem.* **12**, 210.

Fullmer, H. M., and Martin, G. R. (1964). *Nature (London)* **202**, 302.

Gabbiani, G., Tuchweber, B., Côté, G., and LeFort, P. (1968). *Calcif. Tissue Res.* **2**, 30.

Gage, P-W., and Eisenberg, R. S. (1969). *J. Gen. Physiol.* **53**, 265.

Gaillard, P. J. (1959). *Develop. Biol.* **1**, 152.

Gaillard, P. J. (1961). *In* "The Parathyroids" (R. O. Greep and R. V. Talmage, eds.), p. 20. Thomas, Springfield, Illinois.

Galante, L., Gudmundsson, T. V., Matthews, E. W., Tse, A., Williams, E. D., Woodhouse, N. J. Y., and MacIntyre, I. (1968). *Lancet* **2**, 537.

Gallena, A. M., Helmboldt, C. F., Frier, H. J., Nielsen, S. W., and Eaton, H. D. (1970). *J. Nutr.* **100**, 129.

Gardner, W. U., and Pfeiffer, C. A. (1939). *Anat. Rec.* **73**, Suppl. 21.

Garn, S. M., Rohmann, C. G., and Wagner, B. (1967). *Fed. Proc., Fed. Amer. Soc. Exp. Biol.* **26**, 1729.

Gaster, D., Havivi, E., and Guggenheim, K. (1967). *Brit. J. Nutr.* **21**, 413.

Gaunt, W. E., and Irving, J. T. (1940). *J. Physiol. (London)* **99**, 18.

Gaunt, W. E., Griffith, H. D., and Irving, J. T. (1942). *J. Physiol. (London)* **100**, 372.

Gee, A., and Dietz, V. R. (1955). *Anal. Chem.* **77**, 2961.

Gerschberg, H. (1962). *Trans. N.Y. Acad Sci.* [2] **24**, 273.

Gershoff, S. N., Legg, M. A., O'Connor, F. J., and Hegsted, D. M. (1957). *J. Nutr.* **63**, 79.

Giese, W., and Comar, C. L. (1964). *Nature (London)* **202**, 31.

Gilbert, D., and Fenn, W. O. (1957). *J. Gen. Physiol.* **40**, 393.

Gilda, J. E., McCaulay, H. B., and Johansson, E. G. (1943). *J. Dent. Res.* **22**, 200.

Gillman, T., and Wright, L. J. (1966). *Nature (London)* **209**, 263.

Gitelman, H. J., Kukolj, S., and Welt, L. G. (1968). *J. Clin. Invest.* **47**, 118.

Givens, M. H., and Macy, I. G. (1933). *J. Biol. Chem.* **102**, 7.

Gley, E. (1893). *Arch. Anat. Physiol. Physiol. Abt.* [5] **5**, 766.

Glimcher, M. J., and Krane, S. M. (1962). *In* "Radioisotopes and Bone" (P. Lacroix and A. M. Budy, eds) pp. 393–418. Blackwell, Oxford.

Glimcher, M. J., and Krane, S. M. (1964). *Biochim. Biophys. Acta* **90**, 477.

Glimcher, M. J., Hodge, A. J., and Schmitt, F. O. (1957). *Proc. Nat. Acad. Sci. U.S.* **43**, 860.

Glimcher, M. J., Mechanic, G., Bonar, L. C., and Daniel, E. J. (1961). *J. Biol. Chem.* **236**, 3210.

Glimcher, M. J., Freiberg, U. A., and Levine, P. T. (1964a). *Biochem. J.* **93**, 210.

Glimcher, M. J., Mechanic, G. L., and Feiberg, U. A. (1964b). *Biochem. J.* **93**, 198.

Goldman, S. (1960). *In* "Mineral Metabolism" (C. L. Comar and F. Bronner, eds.), Vol. 1, Part 1 A., P. 61. Academic Press, New York.

Goldstein, M., Backstrom, T., Ohi, Y., and Frenkel, R. (1970). *Life Sci.* **9**, 919.

Golub, L., Stern, B., Glimcher, M., and Goldhaber, P. (1968). *Arch. Oral Biol.* **13**, 1395.

Gomez-Puyou, A., de Gomez-Puyou, M. T., Becker, G., and Lehninger, A. L. (1972). *Biochem. Biophys. Res. Commun.* **47**, 814.

Gonzales, F., and Karnovsky, M. J. (1961). *J. Biophys. Biochem. Cytol.* **9**, 299.

Gorlin, R. J., and Chaundry, A. P. (1959). *J. Dent. Res.* **38**, 1008.

Goss, H., and Schmidt, C. L. A. (1930). *J. Biol. Chem.* **86**, 417.

Gould, B. S., and Shwachman, H. (1942). *Amer. J. Physiol.* **135**, 485.

Gould B. S., and Woessner, J. F. (1957). *J. Biol. Chem.* **226**, 289.

Govaerts, J. (1952). *Arch. Int. Physiol.* **60**, 266.

Gran, F. C. (1960). *Acta Physiol. Scand.* **50**, 132.

Gray, T. K., and Munson, P. L. (1969). *Science* **166**, 512.

Greaser, M. L., and Gergely, J. (1971). *J. Gen. Physiol.* **57**, 247.

Green, L. J., Eick, J. D., Miller, W. A., and Leitner, J. W. (1970). *J. Dent. Res.* **49**, 608.

Greenberg, D. M. (1945). *J. Biol. Chem.* **157**, 99.

Greenberg, D. M., and Larson, C. E. (1935) *J. Biol. Chem.* **109**, 105.

Greenberg, D. M., and Miller, W. D. (1941). *J. Nutr.* **22**, 1.

Greenberg, D. M., Boelter, M. D. D., and Knopf, B. W. (1942). *Amer. J. Physiol.* **137**, 459.

Greene, C. H., and Power, M. H. (1931) *J. Biol. Chem.* **91**, 183.

Greeson, C. D., Crawford, E. G., Chandler, D. C., and Bawden, J. W. (1968). *J. Dent. Res.* **47**, 447.

Grette, K. (1962). *Acta Physiol. Scand.* **56**, Suppl. 195, 1.

Greulich, R. C., and Slavkin, H. C. (1965). *Symp. Int. Soc. Cell Biol.* **4**, 199.

Grollman, A. (1927). *J. Biol. Chem.* **72**, 565.

Grollman, A. (1954). *Proc. Soc. Exp. Biol. Med.* **85**, 582.

Gross, J., and Nagai, Y. (1965). *Proc. Nat. Acad. Sci. U.S.* **54**, 1197.

Guri, C. D., and Bernstein, D. S. (1964). *Proc. Soc. Exp. Biol. Med.* **118**, 650.

Guyton, A. C., Coleman, T. G., and Granger, H. J. (1972). *Annu. Rev. Physiol.* **34**, 13.

Haavaldsen, R., and Nicolaysen, R. (1956). *Acta Physiol. Scand.* **36**, 108.

Haddad, J. G., and Chyu, K. J. (1971). *Biochim. Biophys. Acta* **248**, 471.

Hagiwara, S., and Nakajima, S. (1966). *J. Gen. Physiol.* **49**, 807–818.

Hait, H. E. (1967). *Bull. Math. Biophys.* **29**, 319.

Hales, C. N., and Milner, R. D. G. (1968). *J. Physiol. (London)* **199**, 177.

Hall, B. D., Macmillan, D. R., and Bronner, F. (1969). *Amer. J. Clin Nutr.* **22**, 448.

Haller, E. W., Sachs, H., Sperelakis, N., and Share, L. (1965). *Amer. J. Physiol.* **209**, 79.

Hamilton, J. W., and Holdsworth, E. S. (1970). *Biochem. Biophys. Res. Commun.* **40**, 1325.

Hammarström, L. (1967). *Calcif. Tissue Res.* **1**, 229.

Hancox, N. M. (1949). *J. Physiol. (London)* **110**, 205.

Hancox, N. M., and Boothroyd, B. (1961). *J. Biophys. Biochem. Cytol.* **11**, 651.

Hancox, N. M., and Boothroyd, B. (1965). *Clin. Orthop. Related Res.* **40**, 153.

Handelman, C. S., Morse, A., and Irving, J. T. (1964). *Amer. J. Anat.* **115**, 363.

Handler, J. S. (1962). *Amer. J. Physiol.* **202**, 787.

Handler, P., and Cohn, D. V. (1951). *Amer. J. Physiol.* **164**, 646.

Handler, P., Cohn, D. V., and DeMaria, W. J. A. (1951). *Amer. J. Physiol.* **165**, 434.

Hankin, J. H., Margen, S., and Goldsmith, N. F. (1970). *J. Amer. Diet. Ass.* **56**, 212.

Hansard, S. L., and Crowder, H. M. (1957). *J. Nutr.* **62**, 325.

Hansard, S. L., and Plumlee, M. P. (1954). *J. Nutr.* **54**, 17.

Hansard, S. L., Comar, C. L., and Davis, G. K. (1954). *Amer. J. Physiol.* **177**, 383.

Hansel, W., and McEntee, K. (1970). *In* "Duke's Physiology of Domestic Animals" (M. J. Swenson ed.), 8th ed., Chapter 53, p. 1266. Cornell Univ. Press, Ithaca, New York.

Hargis, G. K., Yakulis, V. J., Williams, G. A., and White, A. A. (1964). *Proc. Soc. Exp. Biol. Med.* **117**, 836.

Harmeyer, J., and DeLuca, H. F. (1969). *Arch. Biochem. Biophys.* **133**, 247.

Harper, R. A., and Posner, A. S. (1966). *Proc. Soc. Exp. Biol. Med.* **122**, 137.

Harris, R. S., Baker, N. J., and Nizel, A. E. (1962). *40th Gen. Meet., Int. Ass. Dent. Res.* Abstract No. 145, p. 40.

Harris, W. H., and Heaney, R. P. (1969). *Nature (London)* **223**, 403.

Harrison, D. G., and Long, C. (1968). *J. Physiol. (London)* **199**, 367.

Harrison, G. E., Sutton, A., Shepherd, H., and Widdowson, E. M. (1965). *Brit. J. Nutr.* **19**, 111.

Harrison, H. C., Harrison, H. E., and Park, E. A. (1957). *Proc. Soc. Exp. Biol. Med.* **96**, 768.

Harrison, H. C., Harrison, H. E., and Park, E. A. (1958). *Amer. J. Physiol.* **192**, 432.

Harrison, H. E., and Harrison, H. C. (1942). *Amer. J. Physiol.* **137**, 171.

Harrison, H. E., and Harrison, H. C. (1960). *Amer. J. Physiol.* **199**, 265.

Harrison, H. E., and Harrison, H. C. (1961). *Amer. J. Physiol.* **201**, 1007.

Harrison, H. E., and Harrison, H. C. (1970). *Endocrinology* **86**, 756.

Harrison, J., and McNeill, K. G. (1966). *Nature (London)* **212**, 988.

Harrison, M., and Fraser, R. (1960). *J. Endocrinol.* **21**, 197.

Hart, E. B., Steenbock, H., Hoppert, C. A., Bethke, R. M., and Humphrey, G. C. (1922). *J. Biol. Chem.* **54**, 75.

Hart, E. B., Steenbock, H., Scott, H., and Humphrey, G. C. (1926–1927). *J. Biol. Chem.* **71**, 263.

Hart, H., and Spencer, H. (1967). *Proc. Soc. Exp. Biol. Med.* **126**, 365.

Hart, H. E. (1967). *Bull. Math. Biophys.* **29**, 319.

Hartles, R. L., Leaver, A. G., and Triffitt, J. T. (1964). *Arch. Oral Biol.* **9**, 725.

Hartshorne, D. J., and Mueller, H. (1968). *Biochem. Biophys. Res. Commun.* **31**, 647.

Hashim, G., and Clark, J. (1969). *Biochem. J.* **112**, 275.

Hass, G. M., Trueheart, R. E., Taylor, C. B., and Stumpe, M. (1958). *Amer. J. Pathol.* **34**, 395.

Hasselbach, W. (1957). *Biochim. Biophys. Acta* **25**, 562.

Hasselbach, W. (1964a). *Fed. Proc., Fed. Amer. Soc. Exp. Biol.* **23**, 909.

Hasselbach, W. (1964b). *Progr. Biophys. Mol. Biol.* **14**, 167.

Hasselbach, W., and Makinose, M. (1961). *Biochem. Z.* **333**, 518.

Hasselbach, W., and Makinose, M. (1963). *Biochem. Z.* **339**, 94.

Haury, V. G. (1930). *J. Biol. Chem.* **89**, 467.

Haussler, M. R., and Norman, A. W. (1967). *Arch. Biochem. Biophys.* **118**, 145.

Haussler, M. R., Myrtle, J. F., and Norman, A. W. (1968). *J. Biol. Chem.* **243**, 4055.

Haussler, M. R., Nogade, L. A., and Rasmussen, H. (1970). *Nature (London)* **228**, 1199.

Heaney, R. P., and Whedon, G. D. (1958). *J. Clin. Endocrinol. Metab.* **18**, 1246.

Hebert, L. A., LeMann, J., Petersen, J. R., and Lennon, E. J. (1966). *J. Clin. Invest.* **45**, 1886.

Hegsted, D. M. (1967). *Fed. Proc., Fed. Amer. Soc. Exp. Biol.* **26**, 1747.

Hegsted, D. M., Moscoso, I., and Collazos, C. C. (1952). *J. Nutr.* **46**, 181.

Heilbrunn, L. V., and Wiercinski, F. J. (1947). *J. Cell. Comp. Physiol.* **29**, 15.

Hekkelman, J. W. (1961). *Biochim. Biophys. Acta* **47**, 426.

Heller-Steinberg, M. (1951). *Amer. J. Anat.* **89**, 347.

Hellman, D. E., Au, W. Y. W., and Bartter, F. C. (1965). *Amer. J. Physiol.* **209**, 643.

Hendrickson, H. S., and Fullington, J. G. (1965). *Biochemistry* **4**, 1599.

Henrikson, P. Å., Lutwak, L., Krook, L., Skogerboe, R., Kallfelz, F., Bélanger, L. F., Marier, J. R., Shiffy, B. F., Rananus, B., and Hirsch, C. (1970). *J. Nutr.* **100**, 631.

Herman, H., François, P., and Fabry, C. (1961). *Bull. Soc. Chim. Biol.* **43**, 629.

Herring, G. M. (1964). *Clin. Orthop. Related Res.* **36**, 169.

Herrmann-Eilee, M. P. M. (1964). *J. Histochem. Cytochem.* **12**, 481.

Herrmann-Eilee, M. P. M., and Konijn, T. M. (1970) *Nature (London)* **227**, 177.

Hess, W. C., and Lee, C. (1952). *J. Dent. Res.* **31**, 793.

Hess, W. C., Lee, C. Y., and Neidig, B. A. (1952). *J. Dent. Res.* **31**, 791.

Heubner, W., and Rona, R. (1923). *Biochem. Z.* **135**, 248.

Hiatt, H. H., and Thompson, D. D. (1957). *J. Clin. Invest.* **36**, 557.

Hill, D. K. (1964). *J. Physiol. (London)* **175**, 275.

Hironaka, R., Draper, H. H., and Kastelic, J. (1960). *J. Nutr.* **71**, 356.

Hirsch, P. T., Gauthier, S. F., and Munson, P. L. (1963). *Endocrinology* **73**, 244.

Hirschman, A., and Dziewiatkowski, D. (1966). *Science* **154**, 393.

Hirschman, A., and Silverstein, D. (1968). *Proc. Soc. Exp. Biol. Med.* **129**, 675.

Hodge, A. J., and Petruska, J. A. (1963). *Proc. Int. Symp. Protein Struc. Crystallogr.* (1963) pp. 1–12.

Hodge, H. C. (1938). Quoted in "A Textbook of Dental Histology and Embryology" by F. B. Noyes, I. Schour, and H. J. Noyes. Kimpton, London.

Hodgkin, A. L. (1951). *Biol. Rev. Cambridge Phil. Soc.* **26**, 339.

Hodgkin, A. L., and Huxley, A. F., (1952). *J. Physiol. (London)* **116**, 449.

Hodgkin, A. L., and Katz, B. (1949). *J. Physiol. (London)* **108**, 37.

Hodgkin, A. L., and Keynes, R. D. (1957). *J. Physiol. (London)* **138**, 253.

Hodgkin, A. L., Huxley, A. F., and Katz, B. (1952). *J. Physiol. (London)* **116**, 424.

Hoffman, R. S., Martino, J. A., Wahl, G., and Arky, R. A. (1969). *J. Lab. Clin. Med.* **74**, 915.

Hoffström, K. A. (1910). *Skand. Arch. Physiol.* **23**, 326.

Hogben, C. A. M., and Bollman, J. L. (1951). *Amer. J. Physiol.* **164**, 670.

Hokin, L. E. (1966). *Biochim. Biophys. Acta* **115**, 219.

Holdsworth, E. S. (1965). *Biochem. J.* **96**, 475.

Holdsworth, E. S. (1970). *J. Membrane Biol.* **3**, 43.

Holman, C. A., Mawer, E. B., and Smith, D. J. (1970). *Biochem. J.* **120**, 29P.

Holmes, J. M., Beebe, R. A., Posner, A. S., and Harper, R. A. (1970). *Proc. Soc. Exp. Biol. Med.* **133**, 1250.

Hosoya, N., Watanabe, T., and Fujimori, A. (1964). *Biochim. Biophys. Acta.* **84**, 770.

Howard, J. E. (1954). *In* "Metabolic Interactions" (E. C. Reifenstein, ed.), Trans. 5th Conf., pp. 11–42. Josiah Macy, Jr. Found., New York.

Howard, P. J., Wilde, W. S., and Malvin, R. L. (1959). *Amer. J. Physiol.* **197**, 337.

Howell, D. S., and Carlson, L. (1968). *Exp. Cell Res.* **51**, 185.

Howell, D. S., Marquez, J. F., and Pita, J. C. (1965). *Arthritis Rheum.* **8**, 1039.

Howell, D. S., Pita, J. C., Marquez, J. F., and Madruga, J. E. (1968). *J. Clin. Invest.* **47**, 1121.

Hubbard, J. I., Jones, S. F., and Landau, E. (1968). *J. Physiol. (London)* **196**, 75.

Huffman, C. F., Robinson, C. S., and Winter, O. B. (1930). *J. Dairy Sci.* **13**, 432.

Hulth, A., and Olerud, S. (1963). *Brit. J. Exp. Pathol.* **44**, 491.

Hummel, F. C., Sternberger, H. R., Hunscher, H. A., and Macy, I. G. (1936). *J. Nutr.* **11**, 235.

Humphrey, J. H., and Jaques, R. (1955). *J. Physiol. (London)* **128**, 9.

Hunscher, H. A. (1930). *J. Biol. Chem.* **86**, 37.

Hunt, R. D., Garcia, F. G., Hegsted, D. M , and Kaplinsky, N. (1967). *Science* **157**, 943.

Hurwitz, S. (1968). *Biochim. Biophys. Acta* **156**, 389.

Hurwitz, S., Stacey, R. E., and Bronner, F. (1969) *Amer. J. Physiol.* **216**, 254.

Hurxthal, L. M., and Vose, G. P. (1969). *Calcif. Tissue Res.* **4**, 245.

Hutton, J. J., Tappel, A. L., and Udenfriend, S. (1967). *Arch. Biochem. Biophys.* **118**, 231.

Huxley, A. F., and Peachey, L. D. (1964). *J. Cell Biol.* **23**, 107A.

Huxley, A. F., and Straub, R. W. (1958). *J. Physiol. (London)* **143**, 40P.

Huxley, A. F., and Taylor R. E. (1955). *Nature (London)* **176**, 1068.

Huxley, A. F., and Taylor, R. E. (1958). *J. Physiol. (London)* **144**, 426.

Huxley, H. E. (1964). *Nature (London)* **202**, 1067.

Huxley, H. E. (1971). *15th Annu. Meet., Biophys. Soc. Abstr.* p. 235a.

Hwang, W. S. S., Tonna, E. A., and Cronkite, E. P. (1962). *Nature (London)* **193**, 896.

Ibsen, K. H., and Urist, M. R. (1964). *Nature (London)* **203**, 761.

Imrie, M. H., Neville, P. F., Snellgrove, A. W., and Deluca, H. F. (1967). *Arch. Biochem. Biophys.* **120**, 525.

Iob, V., and Swanson, W. W. (1934). *Amer. J. Dis. Child.* **47**, 302.

Irons, L. I., and Perkins, D. J. (1962). *Biochem. J.* **84**, 152.

Irving, J. T. (1944). *J. Physiol. (London)* **103**, 9.

Irving, J. T. (1946). *J. Physiol. (London)* **105**, 16.

Irving, J. T. (1949). *J. Physiol. (London)* **108**, 92.

Irving, J. T. (1950a). *Brit. J. Exp. Pathol.* **31**, 458.

Irving, J. T. (1950b). *S. Afr. Med. J.* **24**, 601.

Irving, J. T. (1956a). *Med. Klin. (Munich)* **51**, 690.

Irving, J. T. (1956b). *Nature (London)* **178**, 1321.

Irving, J. T. (1957). "Calcium Metabolism," p. 14. Wiley, New York.

Irving, J. T. (1958). *Nature (London)* **181**, 704.

Irving, J. T. (1960). *Clin. Orthop. Related Res.* **17**, 92.

Irving, J. T. (1963). *Arch. Oral Biol.* **8**, 735.

Irving, J. T. (1965). *Arch. Oral Biol.* **10**, 189.

Irving, J. T. (1973). *Arch. Oral Biol.* **18**, 137.

Irving, J. T., and Bond, J. A. (1968). *Amer. J. Anat.* **123**, 119.

Irving, J. T., and Boyle, P. E. (1952). *J. Dent. Res.* **31**, 508.

Irving, J. T., and Durkin, J. F. (1965). *Arch. Oral Biol.* **10**, 179.

Irving, J. T., and Handelman, C. S. (1963). *In* "Mechanisms of Hard Tissue Destruction," Publ. No. 75, p. 515. Amer. Ass. Advan. Sci., Washington, D.C.

Irving, J. T., and Heeley, J. D. (1970a). *Calcif. Tissue Res.* **5**, 64.

Irving, J. T., and Heeley, J. D. (1970b). *Calcif. Tissue Res.* **6**, 254.

Irving, J. T., and Migliore, S. A. (1965). *Amer. J. Anat.* **117**, 151.

Irving, J. T., and Nienaber, M. W. P. (1946). *J. Dent. Res.* **25**, 327.

Irving, J. T., and Richards, M. B. (1939). *Nature (London)* **144**, 908.

Irving, J. T., and Rönning, O. V. (1962). *Arch. Oral Biol.* **7**, 357.

Irving, J. T., and Weinmann, J. P. (1948). *J. Dent. Res.* **27**, 669.

Irving, J. T., and Wuthier, R. E. (1968). *Clin. Orthop. Related Res.* **56**, 237.

Irving, J. T., Schibler, D., and Fleisch, H. (1966). *Proc. Soc. Exp. Biol. Med.* **122**, 852.

Irving, M. H. (1964). *J. Anat.* **98**, 631.

Isaacson, L. C. (1962). *Nature (London)* **196**, 273.

Isaksson, B., and Sjögren, B. (1967). *Proc. Nutr. Soc.* **26**, 106.

Ishida, A. (1967). *Jap. J. Physiol.* **17**, 308.

Ishida, A. (1968). *Jap. J. Physiol.* **18**, 471.

Issekutz, B., Blizzard, J. J., Birkhead, N. C., and Rodahl, K. (1966). *J. Appl. Physiol.* **21**, 1013.

Jacobson, A., Schwartz, M., and Rehm, W. (1965). *Amer. J. Physiol.* **209**, 134.

Jasper, D. (1967). *J. Cell Biol.* **32**, 219.

Jeffay, H., and Boyne, H. R. (1964). *Amer. J. Physiol.* **206**, 415.

Jöbsis F. F., and O'Connor, M. J. (1966). *Biochem. Biophys. Res. Commun.* **25**, 246.

Johansen, E., and Parks, H. F. (1960). *J. Biophys. Biochem. Cytol.* **7**, 743.

Johnston, C. C., Deiss, W. P., and Miner, E. B. (1962). *J. Biol. Chem.* **207**, 3560.

Johnston, C. C., Deiss, W. P., and French, R. S. (1965). *Proc. Soc. Exp. Biol. Med.* **118**, 551

Johnston, F. A., and Folsom, R. A. (1961). *J. Amer. Diet. Ass.* **39**, 220.

Johnston, F. A., Tudwell, C., and Diao, E. (1956). *Fed. Proc., Fed. Amer. Soc. Exp. Biol.* **15**, 559.

Johnston, F. A., Debrock, L., and Diao, E. K. (1958). *Amer. J. Clin. Nutr.* **6**, 136.

Joseph, N. P., Engel, M. B., and Catchpole, H. R. (1953). *Fed. Proc., Fed. Amer. Soc. Exp. Biol.* **12**, 227.

Kallfelz, F. A., Taylor, A. N., and Wasserman, R. H. (1967). *Proc. Soc. Exp. Biol. Med.* **125**, 54.

Kantha, J., Narayanarao, M., Swaminathan, M., and Subrahmanyan, V. (1957). *Brit. J. Nutr.* **11**, 388.

Kashiwa, H. K. (1968). *Anat. Rec.* **162**, 177.

Katchman, B. J. (1961). *In* "Phosphorus and its Compounds" (J. R. Van Wazer, ed.), Vol. II, pp. 1281–1343, Wiley (Interscience), New York.

Katz, B. (1971). *Science* **173**, 123.

Katz, B., and Miledi, R. (1965). *Proc. Roy. Soc., Ser. B.* **161**, 496.

Katz, B., and Miledi, R. (1967a). *Proc. Roy. Soc., Ser. B* **167**, 23.

Katz, B., and Miledi, R. (1967b). *J. Physiol. (London)*, **189**, 535.

Katz, B., and Miledi, R. (1967c). *J. Physiol. (London)* **192**, 407.

Katz, B., and Miledi, R. (1969a). *J. Physiol. (London)* **203**, 689.

Katz, B., and Miledi, R. (1969b). *J. Physiol. (London)* **203**, 459.

Katz, B., and Miledi, R. (1970). *J. Physiol. (London)* **207**, 789.

Katz, J. (1896). *Pfluegers Arch. Gesamte Physiol. Menschen Tiere* **63**, 1.

Kay, H. D. (1928). *J. Physiol. (London)* **65**, 374.

Keating, F. R., Jones, J. D., Elveback, L. R., and Randall, R. V. (1969). *J. Lab. Clin. Med.* **73**, 825.

Kelly, D. E. (1969). *J. Ultrastruct. Res.* **29**, 37.

Kelly, J. S. (1965). *Nature (London)* **205**, 296.

Kenny, A. D., and Heiskell, C. A. (1965). *Proc. Soc. Exp. Biol. Med.* **120**, 269.

Kenny, A. D., Draskóczy, P. R., and Goldhaber, P. (1959). *Amer. J. Physiol.* **197**, 502.

Keutmann, H. T., Aurback, G. D., Dawson, B. F., Niall, H. D., Deftos, L. J., and Potts, J. T., Jr. (1971). *Biochemistry* **10**, 2779.

Keynes, R. D. (1951). *J. Physiol. (London)* **114**, 119.

Keynes, R. D., and Lewis, P. R. (1951). *J. Physiol. (London)* **114**, 151.

Keys, A., Brözek, J., Henschel, A., Mickelson, O., and Taylor, H. L. (1950). "The Biology of Human Starvation," Vol. 1, pp. 533–534. Univ. of Minnesota Press, Minneapolis.

Kibrick, E. A., Becks, H., Marx, W., and Evans, H. M. (1941). *Growth* **5**, 437.

Kimberg, D. V., Schachter, D., and Schenker, H. (1961). *Amer. J. Physiol.* **200**, 1256.

King, J. S., and Boyce, W. H. (1959). *Arch. Biochem. Biophys.* **82**, 455.

Kirschner, N., Sage, H. J., and Smith, W. J. (1967). *Mol. Pharmacol.* **3**, 254.

Kitagawa, S., Yoshimura, J., and Tonomura, Y. (1961). *J. Biol. Chem.* **236**, 902.

Kivirikko, K. J., and Prockop, D. J. (1967). *Arch. Biochem. Biophys.* **118**, 611.

Kleeman, C. R., Bernstein, D., Rockney, R., Dowling, J. T., and Maxwell, M. H. (1961). *In* "The Parathyroids" (R. O. Greep and R. V. Talmage, eds.), p. 353. Thomas, Springfield, Illinois.

Kleeman, C. R., Bohannan, J., Bornstein, D., Ling, S., and Maxwell, M. H. (1964). *Proc. Soc. Exp. Biol. Med.* **115**, 29.

Klein, D. C., and Talmage, R. V. (1968). *Proc. Soc. Exp. Biol. Med.* **127**, 95.

Klein, H., and McCollum, E. V. (1931). *Science* **74**, 662.

Kletzien, S. W. F., Templin, V. M., Steenbock, H., and Thomas, B. H. (1932). *J. Biol. Chem.* **97**, 265.

Kodicek, E., and Ashley, D. R. (1960). *Biochem. J.* **75**, 17p; **76**, 14p.

Kodicek, E., and Thompson, G. A. (1965). *In* "Structure and Function of Connective and Skeletal Tissue" (S. Fitton-Jackson *et al.*, eds.), pp. 369–372. Butterworth, London.

Kodicek, E., Cruickshank, E. M., and Ashley, D. R. (1960). *Biochem. J.* **76**, 15p.

Kodicek, E., Darmady, E. M., and Stranach, F. (1961). *Clin. Sci.* **20**, 185.

Kowarski, S., and Schachter, D. (1969). *J. Biol. Chem.* **244**, 211.

Kraicer, J., Milligan, J. V., Gosbee, J. L., Conrad, R. G., and Branson, C. M. (1969). *Endocrinology*, **85**, 1144.

Krane, S. M., Brownell, G. L., Stanbury, J. B., and Corrigan, H. (1956). *J. Clin. Invest.* **35**, 874.

Krane, S. M., Stone, M. J., and Glimcher, M. J. (1965). *Biochim. Biophys. Acta* **97**, 77.

Krane, S. M., Muñoz, A. J., and Harris, E. D. (1970). *J. Clin. Invest.* **49**, 716.

Krawitt, E. L., and Kunin, A. S. (1971). *Proc. Soc. Exp. Biol. Med.* **136**, 530.

Krehl, W. A., and Winters, R. W. (1950). *J. Amer. Diet. Ass.* **26**, 966.

Kreitzman, S. N., and Fritz, M. E. (1970). *J. Dent. Res.* **49**, 1509.

Krishna Rao, G. V. G. (1961). *Nature (London)* **192**, 269.

Kronfeld, D. S., Ramberg, C. F., and Delivoria-Papadoupoulos, M. (1971). *In* "Cellular Mechanism for Calcium Transfer and Homeostasis" (G. Nichols, Jr. and R. H. Wasserman, eds.), pp. 339–349. Academic Press, New York.

Kumamato, Y., and Leblond, C. P. (1956). *J. Dent. Res.* **35**, 147.

Kumamato, Y., and Leblond, C. P. (1958). *J. Dent. Res.* **37**, 147.

Kunin, A. S., and Krane, S. M. (1965a). *Biochim. Biophys. Acta* **107**, 203.

Kunin, A. S., and Krane, S. M. (1965b). *Biochim. Biophys. Acta* **111**, 32.

Kyes, P., and Potter, T. S. (1934). *Anat. Rec.* **60**, 377.

Lamm, M., and Neuman, W. F. (1958). *AMA Arch. Pathol.* **66**, 204.

Landsberg, E. (1915). *Z. Geburts. Cynäk.* **76**, 53.

Lanford, C. S., Campbell, H. L., and Sherman, H. C. (1941). *J. Biol. Chem.* **137**, 627.

Lapière, C. M., Onkelinx, C., and Richelle, L. J. (1965). *In* "Biochimie et physiologie du tissue conjonctif" (P. Comte, ed.), p. 505 Imprimerie Sud, Lyon, France.

Laron, Z., and Boss, J. H. (1962). *Arch. Pathol.* **73**, 26.

Laron, Z., Canlas, B. D., and Crowford, J. D. (1958a). *AMA Arch. Pathol.* **65**, 403.

Laron, Z., Muhlethaler, J. P., and Klein, R. (1958b). *AMA Arch. Pathol.* **65**, 125.

Lassiter, W. E., Gottschalk, C. W., and Mylle, M. (1963). *Amer. J. Physiol.* **204**, 771.

Lawson, D. E. M., Wilson, P. W., and Kodicek, E. (1969a). *Nature (London)* **222**, 171.

Lawson, D. E. M., Wilson, P. W., and Kodicek, E. (1969b). *Biochem. J.* **115**, 269.

Lawson, D. E. M., Fraser, D. R., Kodicek, E., Morris, H. R., and Williams, D. H. (1971). *Nature (London)* **228**, 230.

Leach, A. A. (1958). *Biochem. J.* **69**, 429.

Leblanc, P., Bourdain, M., and Clauser, H. (1970). *Biochem. Biophys. Res. Commun.* **40**, 754.

Lee, N. M., Wiedemann, I., and Kun, E. (1971). *FEBS Lett.* **18**, 81.

Lefkowitz, R., Roth, J., and Pastan, I. (1970). *Nature (London)* **228**, 864.

Lehman, W., Kendrick-Jones, J., and Szent-Györgyi, A. G. (1970). *J. Mol. Biol.* **54**, 313.

Lehninger, A. L. (1949). *J. Biol. Chem.* **178**, 625.

Lehninger, A. L. (1970). *Biochem. J.* **119**, 129.

Lehninger, A. L., Carafoli, E., and Rossi, C. S. (1967). *Advan. Encymol.* **29**, 259.

Leitch, I. (1936–1937). *Nutr. Abstr. Rev.* **6**, 553.

Lekan, E. C., Laskin, D. M., and Engel, M. B. (1960). *Amer. J. Physiol.* **199**, 856.

Lengemann, F. W. (1959). *J. Nutr.* **69**, 23.

Lengemann, F. W., and Comar, C. L. (1963). *J. Nutr.* **81**, 95.

Lengemann, F. W., and Dobbins, J. W. (1958). *J. Nutr.* **66**, 45.

Lengemann, F. W., Wasserman, R. H., and Comar, C. L. (1959). *J. Nutr.* **68**, 443.

Levinskas, G. (1953). Doctoral Thesis, University of Rochester, Rochester, New York.

Levinsky, N. G., and Davidson, D. G. (1957). *Amer. J. Physiol.* **191**, 530.

Likins, R. C., Bavetta, L. A., and Posner, A. S. (1957). *Arch. Biochem. Biophys.* **70**, 401.

Liljestrand, A., and Swedin, B. (1952). *Acta Physiol. Scand.* **25**, 168.

Linder, G. C. (1940). *Biochem. J.* **34**, 1574.

Loewenstein, W. R. (1967a). *Develop. Biol.* **15**, 503.

Loewenstein, W. R. (1967b). *J. Colloid Interface Sci.* **25**, 34.

Logan, M. A., and Taylor, H. L. (1938). *J. Biol. Chem.* **125**, 391.

Loken, H. F., Havel, R. J., Gordan, G. S., and Whittington, S. L. (1960). *J. Biol. Chem.* **235**, 3654.

Long, C., and Mouat, B. (1971). *Biochem. J.* **123**, 829.

Longson, D., Mills, J. N., Thomas, S., and Yates, P. A. (1956). *J. Physiol. (London)* **131**, 555.

Lorch, I. (1947). *Quart. J. Microsc. Sci.* **88**, 367.

Lough, S. A., Rivera, J., and Comar, C. L. (1963). *Proc. Soc. Exp. Biol. Med.* **112**, 631.

Lucy, J. A., Dingle, J. T., and Fell, H. B. (1961). *Biochem. J.* **79**, 500.

Lueker, C. E., and Lofgreen, G. P. (1961). *J. Nutr.* **74**, 233.

Luick, J. R., Boda, J. M., and Kleiber, M. (1957). *J. Nutr.* **61**, 597.

Lutwak, L., and Shapiro, J. R. (1964). *Science* **144**, 1155.

McAleese, D. M., and Forbes, R. M. (1961). *J. Nutr.* **73**, 94.

McCance, R. A., and Widdowson, E. M. (1943). *Lancet* **1**, 1230.

McClure, F. J., and McCann, H. G. (1960). *Arch. Oral Biol.* **2**, 151.

McClure, F. J., and Miller, A. (1959). *J. Dent. Res.* **38**, 776.

McCollum, E. V., Simmonds, N., Becker, J. E., and Shipley, P. G. (1922). *J. Biol. Chem.* **53**, 293.

McConnell, D. (1955). *Biochim. Biophys. Acta* **17**, 450.

McConnell, D. (1960). *Arch. Oral Biol.* **3**, 28.

McConnell, D., Frajola, W. D., and Deamer, D. W. (1961). *Science* **133**, 281.

McCullagh, E. P., and McCullagh, D. R. (1932). *J. Lab. Clin. Med.* **17**, 754.

MacDonald, N. S., Hitchinson, D. L., Hepler, M., and Flynn, E. (1965). *Proc. Soc. Exp. Biol. Med.* **119**, 476.

McElligott, T. F. (1962). *J. Pathol. Bacteriol.* **83**, 347.

MacGregor, J. (1964). *In* "Bone and Tooth" (H. J. J. Blackwood, ed.), pp. 351–355 Pergamon, Oxford.

MacGregor, J., and Brown, W. E. (1965). *Nature (London)* **205**, 359.

MacGregor, J., Nordin, B. E. C., and Robertson, W. G. (1965). *Nature (London)* **207**, 861.

MacGregor, R. R., Hamilton, J. W., and Cohn, D. V. (1970). *Biochim. Biophys. Acta* **222**, 482.

MacIntyre, I., Boss, S., and Troughton, V. A. (1963). *Nature (London)* **198**, 1058.

Mack, P. B., and LaChance, P. L. (1967). *Amer. J. Clin. Nutr.* **20**, 1194.

McLean, F. C., and Hastings, A. B. (1935a). *Amer. J. Med. Sci.* **189**, 601.

McLean, F. C., and Hastings, A. B. (1935b). *J. Biol. Chem.* **108**, 285.

McLean, F. C., and Hinrichs, M. A. (1938). *Amer. J. Physiol.* **121**, 580.

McLean, F. C., and Urist, M. R. (1955) "Bone, an Introduction to the Physiology of Skeletal Tissues," 1st ed. University of Chicago Press, Chicago, Illinois.

McLean, F. C., and Urist, M. R. (1968). "Bone, an Introduction to the Physiology of Skeletal Tissues," 3rd ed. Univ. of Chicago Press, Chicago, Illinois.

McLean, F. C., Lipton, M. A., Bloom, W., and Barrón, E. S. G. (1946). *In* "Metabolic Aspects of Convalescence" (E. C. Reifenstein, ed.), Trans. 14th Conf., pp. 9–19. Josiah Macy, Jr. Found., New York.

Macomber, D. (1927). *J. Amer. Med. Ass.* **88**, 6.

Pharmacol. **17**, 241.

Makinose, M. (1969). *Eur. J. Biochem.* **10**, 74.

Makinose, M., and Hasselbach, W. (1965). *Biochem. Z.* **343**, 360.

Makinose, M., and Hasselbach, W. (1971). *FEBS Lett.* **12**, 271.

Malamed, S., Poisner, A. M., Trifaro, J. M., and Douglas, W. W. (1968). *Biochem.*

Mallon, M. G., Jordon, R., and Johnson, M. (1930). *J. Biol. Chem.* **88**, 163.

Malm, O. J. (1953). *Scand. J. Clin. Lab. Invest.* **5**, 75.

Mankin, H. J. (1964). *J. Bone Joint Surg., Amer. Vol.* **46**, 1253.

Mankin, H. J., and Lippiello, L. (1969). *J. Bone Joint Surg., Amer. Vol.* **51**, 862.

Manners, M. J., and McCrea, M. R. (1963). *Brit. J. Nutr.* **17**, 495.

Månsson-Angmar, B. (1971). *Arch. Oral Biol.* **16**, 135.

Marino, A. A., and Becker, R. O. (1967). *Nature (London)* **213**, 697.

Markwardt, F., and Barthel, W. (1964). *Naunyn-Schmiedebergs Arch. Pharmakol. Exp. Pathol.* **249**, 176.

Markwardt, F., Barthel, W., Hoffmann, A., and Wittier, E. (1965), *Naunyn-Schmiedebergs Arch. Pharmacol. Exp. Pathol.* **251**, 255.

Marsh, B. B. (1951). *Nature (London)* **167**, 1065.

Marsh, B. B. (1952). *Biochim. Biophys. Acta* **9**, 247.

Marshall, J. H. (1969). *In* "Mineral Metabolism" (C. L. Comar and F. Bronner, eds.), Vol. 3, Chapter 1, p. 1. Academic Press, New York.

Martin, D. L., Melancon, M. J., and DeLuca, H. F. (1969). *Biochem. Biophys. Res Commun.* **35**, 819.

Martin, G. R., Schiffmann, E., Bladen, H. A., and Nylen, M. (1963). *J. Cell Biol.* **16**, 243.

Martin, J. H., and Matthews, J. L. (1969). *Calcif. Tissue Res.* **3**, 184.

Martin, N. H., and Perkins, D. J. (1950). *Biochem. J.* **47**, 323.

Martin, N. H., and Perkins, D. J. (1953). *Biochem. J.* **54**, 643.

Martonosi, A. (1967). *Biochem. Biophys. Res. Commun.* **29**, 753.

Martonosi, A. (1969). *J. Biol. Chem.* **244**, 613.

Martonosi, A. (1971). *In* "Biomembranes" (L. A. Manson, ed), Vol. 1, p. 191. Plenum, New York.

Martonosi, A., and Feretos, R. (1964). *J. Biol. Chem.* **239**, 659.

Martonosi, A., Donley, J. R., and Halpin, R. A. (1968). *J. Biol. Chem.* **243**, 61.

Massry, S. G., Coburn, J. W., Chapman, L. W., and Kleeman, C. R. (1968a). *J. Lab. Clin. Med.* **71**, 212.

Massry, S. G., Coburn, J. W., Chapman, L. W., and Kleeman, C. R. (1968b) *Amer. J. Physiol.* **214**, 1403.

Massry, S. G., Ahumada, J. J., Coburn, J. W., and Kleeman, C. R. (1970). *Amer. J. Physiol.* **219**, 881.

Matthews, E. K. (1970). *In* "Calcium and Cellular Function" (A. W. Cuthbert, ed.), p. 163. St. Martin's Press, New York.

Matthews, J. L., Martin, J. H., and Collins, E. J. (1968). *Clin. Orthop. Related Res.* **58**, 213.

Matthews, J. L., Martin, J. H., Sampson, H. W., Kunin, A. S., and Roan, J. H. (1970). *Calcif. Tissue Res.* **5**, 91.

Matukas, V. J., and Krikos, G. A. (1968). *J. Cell Biol.* **39**, 43.

Mawer, E. B., and Stanbury, S. W. (1968). *Biochem. J.* **110**, 53P.

Mayer, G. P. Marshak, R. R., and Kronfeld, D. S. (1966). *Amer. J. Physiol.* **211**, 1366.

Mayer, G. P., Ramberg, C. F., and Kronfeld, D. S. (1967). *J. Nutr.* **92**, 253.

Mayer, G. P., Ramberg, C. F., and Kronfeld, D. S. (1968). *J. Nutr.* **95**, 202.

Maynard, L. A., Boggs, D., Fisk, G., and Segum, D. (1958). *J. Nutr.* **64**, 85.

Mears, D. C. (1969). *Exp. Cell Res.* **58**, 427.

Mecca, C. E., Martin, G. R., and Goldhaber, P. (1963). *Proc. Soc. Exp. Biol. Med.* **113**, 538.

Meintzer, R. B., Nelson, D. R., and Freeman, S. (1961). *Amer. J. Physiol.* **201**, 531.

Melancon, M. J., and DeLuca, H. F. (1970). *Biochemistry* **9**, 1659.

Mellanby, E. (1947). *J. Physiol. (London)* **105**, 352.

Mendelsohn, L. (1962). *J. Nutr.* **77**, 198.

Menkin, V., Wolbach, S. B., and Menkin, M. F. (1934). *Amer. J. Pathol.* **10**, 569.

Meredith, H. V. (1941). *Amer. J. Phys. Anthropol.* **28**, 1.

Meyer, D. L., and Forbes, R. M. (1968). *Proc. Soc. Exp. Biol. Med.* **128**, 157.

Meyer, J., Bolen, R. J., and Antin, J. (1959). *Arch. Biochem. Biophys.* **81**, 340.

Meyer, W. L., and Kunin, A. S. (1969). *Arch. Biochem. Biophys.* **129**, 438.

Michelakis, A. M. (1970). *Proc. Soc. Exp. Biol. Med.* **135**, 13.

Miledi, R. (1966). *Nature (London)* **212**, 1233.

Milhaud, G. (1965). *Proc. Int. Endocrine Congr. 2nd, 1964* Vol. 2 p. 912.

Milhaud, G., and Moukhtar, M. S. (1966). *Nature (London)* **211**, 1186.

Milhaud, G., Perault, A. M., and Moukhtar, M. S. (1965). *C. R. Acad. Sci.* **261**, 813.

Miller, A., and Tregear, R. T. (1970). *Nature (London)* **226**, 1060.

Miller, E. J., Epstein, E. H., and Piez, K. A. (1971). *Biochem. Biophys. Res. Commun.* **42**, 1024.

Miller, E. R., Ullrey, D. E., Zutant, C. L., Baltzer, B. V., Schmidt, D. A., Hoefer, J. A., and Levecke, R. W. (1962). *J. Nutr.* **77**, 7.

Mitchell, H. H., and Curzon, E. G. (1939). "The Dietary Requirement of Calcium and its Significance." Hermann, Paris.

Mitchell, H. H., Hamilton, T. S., Steggerda, F. R., and Bean, H. W. (1945). *J. Biol. Chem.* **158**, 625.

Mitchell, P (1966). "Chemiosmotic Coupling in Oxidative and Photosynthetic Phosphorylation." Glynn Res. Ltd., Bodmin, Cornwall, England.

Mitchell, P., and Moyle, J. (1965a). *Nature (London)* **208**, 147.

Mitchell, P., and Moyle, J. (1965b). *Nature (London)* **208**, 1205.

Molnar, Z. (1959). *J. Ultrastruct. Res.* **3**, 39.

Molnar, Z. (1960). *Clin. Orthop.* **17**, 38.

Mongar, J. L., and Schild, H. O. (1962). *Physiol. Rev.* **42**, 226.

Moore, E. W. (1970). *J. Clin. Invest.* **49**, 318.

Moore, L. A. (1939). *J. Nutr.* **17**, 443.

Moore, L. A., Huffman, C. F., and Duncan, C. W. (1935). *J. Nutr.* **9**, 533.

Moore, T., and Wang, Y. L. (1945). *Biochem. J.* **39**, 222.

Moore, T., Impey, S. G., Martin, P. E. N., and Symonds, K. R. (1963). *J. Nutr.* **80**, 162.

Morgareidge, K., amd Manley, M. L. (1939). *J. Nutr.* **18**, 411.

Morii, H., and DeLuca, H. F. (1967). *Amer. J. Physiol.* **213**, 358.

Morii, H., Lund, J., Neville, P. F., and DeLuca, H. F. (1967). *Arch. Biochem. Biophys.* **120**, 508.

Morris, E. R., and O'Dell, B. L. (1963). *J. Nutr.* **81**, 175.

Morse, A., and Greep, R. O. (1951). *Anat. Rec.* **111**, 193.

Moseley, J. M., Matthews, E. W., Breed, R. H., Galante, L., Tse, A., and MacIntyre, I. (1968). *Lancet* **1**, 108.

Moss, D. W., Eaton, R. H., Smith, J. K., and Whitley, L. G. (1967). *Biochem. J.* **102**, 53.

Muller, S. A., Posner, A. S., and Firschein, H. E. (1966). *Proc. Soc. Exp. Biol. Med.* **121**, 844.

Munday, K. A., Ansari, A. Q., Oldroyd, D., and Akhtar, M. (1968). *Biochim. Biophys. Acta* **166**, 748.

Munson, P. L., and Gray, T. K. (1969). *Science* **166**, 512.

Murad, F., Brewer, H. B., and Vaughan, M. (1970). *Proc. Nat. Acad. Sci. U.S.* **65**, 446.

Myers, H. M., and Engström, A. (1965). *Exp. Cell Res.* **40**, 182.

Myrtle, J. F., Haussler, M. R., and Norman, A. W. (1970). *J. Biol. Chem.* **245**, 1190.

Nagai, T., Makinose, M., and Hasselbach, W. (1960). *Biochim. Biophys. Acta* **43**, 223.

Nagata, N., and Rasmussen, H. (1968). *Biochemistry* **7**, 3728.

Nagata, N., and Rasmussen, H. (1970). *Proc. Nat. Acad. Sci. U.S.* **65**, 368.

Nash, H. A., and Tobias, J. M. (1964). *Proc. Nat. Acad. Sci. U.S.* **51**, 476.

Neer, R., Berman, M., Fisher, L., and Rosenberg, L. E. (1967). *J. Clin. Invest.* **46**, 1364.

Nelson, M. M., Sulon, E., Becks, H., Wainwright, W. W., and Evans, H. M. (1947). *Proc. Soc. Exp. Biol. Med.* **66**, 631.

Nelson, M. M., Sulon, E., Becks, H., Wainwright, W. W., and Evans, H. M. (1950). *Proc. Soc. Exp. Biol. Med.* **73**, 31.

Neuman, W. F., and Mulryan, B. J. (1967). *Calcif. Tissue Res.* **1**, 94.

Neuman, W. F., and Mulryan, B. J. (1968). *Calcif. Tissue Res.* **2**, 237.

Neuman, W. F., and Mulryan, B. J. (1971). *Calcif. Tissue Res.* **7**, 133.

Neuman, W. F., and Neuman, M. W. (1953). *Chem. Rev.* **53**, 1.

Neuman, W. F., and Neuman, M. W. (1958). "The Chemical Dynamics of Bone Mineral." Univ. of Chicago Press, Chicago, Illinois.

Neuman, W. F., Terepka, A. R., Canas, F., and Triffitt, J. T. (1968). *Calcif. Tissue Res.* **2**, 262.

Neville, E., and Holdsworth, E. S. (1968). *Biochim. Biophys. Acta* **163**, 362.

Nicholls, L., and Nimalasuriya, A. (1939). *J. Nutr.* **18**, 563.

Nichols, G. (1963). *In* "Mechanisms of Hard Tissue Destruction," Publ. No. 75, pp. 557–575. Amer. Ass. Advan. Sci. Washington, D.C.

Nichols, G., Schartum, S., and Vaes, G. M. (1963). *Acta Physiol. Scand.* **57**, 51.

Nicholson, T. F. (1959). *Can. J. Biochem. Physiol.* **37**, 113.

Nicholson, T. F., and Shepherd, G. W. (1959). *Can. J. Biochem. Physiol.* **37**, 103.

Nicolaysen, R. (1943). *Acta Physiol. Scand.* **5**, 200.

Nicolaysen, R., Eeg-Larsen, N., and Malm, O. J. (1953). *Physiol. Rev.* **33**, 424.

Niedergerke, R. (1955). *J. Physiol. (London)* **128**, 12P.

Nisbet, J. A., Helliwell, S., and Nordin, B. E. C. (1970). *Clin. Orthop. Related Res.* **70**, 220.

Noble, H. M., and Matty, A. J. (1967). *J. Endocrinol.* **37**, 1117.

Nordin, B. E. C. (1962). *Amer. J. Clin. Nutr.* **10**, 384.

Nordin, B. E. C. (1964). "The Relation between Dietary Calcium and Osteoporosis in Different Parts of the World." Report to Nutrition Section of WHO, Glasgow (privately printed).

Nordin, B. E. C., Glass, H., Smith, D., MacGregor, J., Nesbet, J., and Burns, H. G. (1964). *Tech. Rep. Ser. Int. At. Energy Ag.* **32**, 75–86.

Norman, A. W. (1965). *Science* **149**, 184.

Norman, A. W. (1966). *Biochem. Biophys. Res. Commun.* **23**, 335.

Norman, A. W. (1967). *Clin. Orthop. Related Res.* **52**, 249.

Norman, A. W., and DeLuca, H. F. (1964a). *Biochem. J.* **91**, 124.

Norman, A. W., and DeLuca, H. F. (1964b). *Arch. Biochem. Biophys.* **107**, 69.

Norman, A. W., Mitcheff, A. K., Adams, T. H., and Spielvogel, A. (1970). *Biochim. Biophys. Acta* **215**, 348.

Norman, A. W., Midgett, R. J., Myrtle, J. F., and Nowicki, H. G. (1971a). *Biochem. Biophys. Res. Commun.* **42**, 1082.

Norman, A. W., Myrtle, J. F., Midgett, R. J., Nowicki, H. G., Williams, V., and Popják, G. (1971b). *Science* **173**, 51.

Nylen, M. U., Eanes, E. D., and Omnel, K.-Å. (1963). *J. Cell Biol.* **18**, 109.

Oberst, F. W., and Plass, E. D. (1940). *Amer. J. Obstet. Gynecol.* **40**, 399.

O'Dell, B. L., Morris, E. R., and Regan, W. O. (1960). *J. Nutr.* **70**, 103.

Olsen, E. B., and DeLuca, H. F. (1969). *Science* **165**, 405.

O'Riordan, J. L. H., and Aubach, G. D. (1968). *Endocrinology* **82**, 377.

Owen, E. C., Irving, J. T., and Lyall, A. (1939). *Acta Med. Scand.* **103**, 235.

Ozawa, E., Hosoi, K., and Ebashi, S. (1967). *J. Biochem. (Tokyo)* **61**, 531.

Paegle, R. D. (1966). *Arch. Pathol.* **82**, 474.

Page, S. (1965). *J. Cell Biol.* **26**, 477.

Pak, C. Y., Zisman, E., Evens, R., Jowsey, J., DeLea, C. S., and Bartter, F. C. (1969). *Amer. J. Med.* **47**, 7.

Palade, G. E., and Palay, S. L. (1954). *Anat. Rec.* **118**, 335.

Papworth, D. G., and Patrick, G. (1970). *J. Physiol. (London)* **210**, 999.

Park, E. A. (1939). *Bull. N. Y. Acad. Med.* [2] **15**, 495.

Parsons, J. A. (1969). *Amer. J. Physiol.* **217**, 1599.

Parsons, V., Veall, N., and Butterfield, W. J. H. (1968). *Calcif. Tissue Res.* **2**, 83.

Patriarca, P., and Carafoli, E. (1969). *Experientia* **25**, 598.

Patrick, G. (1970). *J. Physiol. (London)* **207**, 38P.

Payne, J. M., and Sansom, B. F. (1963). *J. Physiol. (London)* **168**, 554.

Payne, J. M., and Sansom, B. F. (1966). *J. Physiol. (London)* **184**, 433.

Pearse, A. G. E., and Tremblay, G. (1958). *Nature (London)* **181**, 1532.

Pease, D. C., Jenden, D. J., and Howell, J. N. (1965). *J. Cell. Comp. Physiol.* **65**, 141.

Pellegrino, E. D., and Biltz, R. M. (1968). *Nature (London)* **219**, 1261.

Perdok, W. G., and Gustafson, G. (1961). *Arch. Oral Biol.* **4**, 70.

Perkin, A. B., Bader, H. I., Tashjian, A. H., and Goldhaber, P. (1968). *Proc. Soc. Exp. Biol. Med.* **128**, 218.

Perris, A. D., Whitfield, J. F., and Rixon, R. H. (1967). *Radiat. Res.* **32**, 550.

Perry, S. V., and Grey, T. C. (1956). *Biochem. J.* **64**, 5P.

Peterson, O. H., Poulsen, J. H., and Thorn, N. A. (1967). *Acta Physiol. Scand.* **71**, 203.

Phang, J. M., Berman, M., Finerman, G. A., Neer, R. M., Rosenberg, L. E., and Hahn, T. J. (1969). *J. Clin. Invest.* **48**, 67.

Philippu, A., and Schümann, H. J. (1962). *Experientia* **18**, 138.

Piez, K. A., Eigner, E. A., and Lewis, M. S. (1963). *Biochemistry* **2**, 58.

Pincus, J. B., Natelson, S., and Lugovoy, J. K. (1951). *Proc. Soc. Exp. Biol. Med.* **78**, 24.

Pletscher, A., Da Prada, M., and Tranzer, J. P. (1968). *Experientia* **24**, 1202.

Poisner, A. M., and Trifaro, J. M. (1967). *Mol. Pharmacol.* **3**, 561.

Ponchon, G., and DeLuca, H. F. (1969). *J. Clin. Invest.* **48**, 1273.

Ponlot, R. (1960). "Le radiocalcium dans l'étude des os," p. 55. Editions Arscia, Brussels.

Popovici, A., Geschickter, C. F., Reinovsky, A., and Rubin, M. (1950). *Proc. Soc. Exp. Biol. Med.* **74**, 415.

Porter, K. R. (1961). *J. Biophys. Biochem. Cytol.* **10**, Suppl., 219.

Porter, K. R., and Palade, G. E. (1957). *J. Biophys. Biochem. Cytol.* **3**, 269.

Posner, A. S. (1969). *Physiol. Rev.* **49**, 760.

Posner, A. S., and Perloff, A. (1957). *J. Res. Nat. Bur. Stand., Sect. A* **58**, 279.

Poulos, P. P. (1957). *J. Lab. Clin. Med.* **49**, 253.

Prockop, D. J., and Kivirikko, K. I. (1968). *In* "Treatise on Collagen" (B. S. Gould, ed.), Vol. 2, Part A, Chapter 5, pp. 215–246. Academic Press, New York.

Pugliarello, M. C., Vittur, F., deBernard, B., Bonucci, E., and Ascenzi, A. (1970). *Calcif. Tissue Res.* **5**, 108.

Puschett, J. B., and Goldberg, M. (1969). *J. Lab. Clin. Med.* **73**, 956.

Rahill, W. J., and Walser, M. (1965). *Amer. J. Physiol.* **208**, 1165.

Raisz, L. G. (1963a). *Nature (London)* **197**, 1015.

Raisz, L. G. (1963b). *Nature (London)* **197**, 1115.

Raisz, L. G. (1965). *Proc. Soc. Exp. Biol. Med.* **119**, 614.

Raisz, L. G. (1967). *Biochim. Biophys. Acta* **148**, 460.

Raisz, L. G., and Hammack, D. F. (1959). *Proc. Soc. Exp. Biol. Med.* **100**, 411.

Raisz, L. G., and O'Brien, J. E. (1963). *Amer. J. Physiol.* **205**, 816.

Raisz, L. G., O'Brien, J. E., and Au, W. Y. W. (1965). *Proc. Soc. Exp. Biol. Med.* **119**, 1048.

Ramberg, C. F., Phang, J. M., and Kronfeld, D. S. (1970). *In* "Parturient Hypocalcemia" (J. J. B. Anderson, ed.), p. 119. Academic Press, New York.

Rasmussen, H. (1970). *Science* **170**, 404.

Rasmussen, H., and Westall, R. G. (1956). *Nature (London)* **178**, 1173.

Rasmussen, H., Waldorf, A., Dziewiatkowski, D. D., and DeLuca, H. F. (1963). *Biochim. Biophys. Acta* **75**, 250.

Rasmussen, H., Arnaud, C., and Hawker, C. (1964). *Science* **144**, 1019.

Rasmussen, H., Chance, B., and Ogata, E. (1965). *Proc. Nat. Acad. Sci U.S.* **53**, 1069.

Rasmussen, H., Schirasu, H., Ogata, E., and Hawker, C. (1967). *J. Biol. Chem.* **242**, 4669.

Rasmussen, H., Pechet, M., and Fast, D. (1968). *J. Clin. Invest.* **47**, 1843.

Rasmussen, P. (1969). *Arch. Oral Biol.* **14**, 1293.

Rasmussen, P. (1970). *Brit. J. Nutr.* **24**, 29.

Raven, A. M., Lengemann, F. W., and Wasserman, R. H. (1960). *J. Nutr.* **72**, 29.

Reaven, G., Schneider, A., and Reaven, E. (1959). *Proc. Soc. Exp. Biol. Med.* **102**, 70.

Reddy, B. S., Pleasants, J. R., and Wostmann, B. S. (1969). *J. Nutr.* **99**, 353.

Reid, J. M., Lutwak, L., and Whedon, G. D. (1968). *J. Amer. Diet. Ass.* **53**, 342.

Reifenstein, E. C., Kinsell, L. W., and Albright, F. (1946). *J. Clin. Endocrinol.* **6**, 470.

Retief, D. H., Cleaton-Jones, P. E., and Turkstra, J. (1970). *J. Dent. Ass. S. Afr.* **25**, 188.

Revel, J. P., and Hay, E. D. (1963). *Z. Zellforsch. Mikrosk. Anat.* **61**, 110.

Reynafarje, B., and Lehninger, A. L. (1969). *J. Biol. Chem.* **244**, 584.

Reynolds, J. J., and Dingle, J. T. (1970). *Calcif. Tissue Res.* **4**, 339.

Rich, C., and Ivanovich, P. (1965). *Ann. Intern. Med.* **63**, 1069.

Richelle, L. J., and Bronner, F. (1963). *Biochem. Pharmacol.* **12**, 647.

Richelle, L. J., and Onkelinx, C. (1969). *In* "Mineral Metabolism" (C. L. Comar and F. Bronner, eds.), Vol. 3, p. 123. Academic Press, New York.

Riddle, O., and McDonald, M. R. (1945). *Endocrinology* **36**, 48.

Riddle, O., and Reinhart, W. H. (1926). *Amer. J. Physiol.* **76**, 660.

Rigal, W. M. (1964). *Proc. Soc. Exp. Biol. Med.* **117**, 794.

Riggs, B. L., Jowsey, J., Kelly, P. J., Jones, J. D., and Maher, F. T. (1969). *J. Clin. Invest.* **48**, 1065.

Rikkers, H., and DeLuca, H. F. (1967). *Amer. J. Physiol.* **213**, 380.

Rikkers, H., Kletziens, R., and DeLuca, H. F. (1969). *Proc. Soc. Exp. Biol. Med.* **130**, 1321.

Robertson, J. D. (1941). *Lancet* **2**, 129.

Robertson, W. V. B. (1950). *J. Biol. Chem.* **187**, 673.

Robinson, R. A., and Watson, M. L. (1952). *Anat. Rec.* **114**, 383.

Robinson, R. A., and Watson, M. L. (1955). *Ann. N.Y. Acad. Sci.* **60**, 596.

Robison, R. (1923). *Biochem. J.* **17**, 286.

Robison, R., McLeod, M., and Rosenheim, A. H. (1930). *Biochem. J.* **24**, 1927.

Rolle, G. K. (1965). *Arch. Oral Biol.* **10**, 393.

Rolle, G. K. (1969). *Calcif. Tissue Res.* **3**, 142.

Romero, P. J., and Whittam, R. (1971). *J. Physiol. (London)* **214**, 481.

Rönnholm, E. (1962a). *J. Ultrastruct. Res.* **6**, 249.

Rönnholm, E. (1962b). *J. Ultrastruct. Res.* **6**, 368.

Rosser, H., Boyde, A., and Stewart, A. D. G. (1967). *Arch. Oral Biol.* **12**, 431.

Rossi, C. S., and Lehninger, A. L. (1963). *Biochem. Z.* **338**, 698.

Rossi, C. S., and Lehninger, A. L. (1964). *J. Biol. Chem.* **239**, 3971.

Rossi, C. S., Bielawski, J., and Lehninger, A. L. (1966). *J. Biol. Chem.* **241**, 1919.

Roth, S. I., Au, W. Y. W., Kunin, A. S., Krane, S. M., and Raisz, L. G. (1968). *Amer. J. Pathol.* **53**, 631.

Rottensten, K. V. (1938). *Biochem. J.* **32**, 1285.

Rowland, R. E. (1966). *Clin. Orthop. Related Res.* **49**, 233.

Rowles, S. L. (1958). *Biochem. J.* **69**, 13p.

Rubin, R. P. (1969). *J. Physiol. (London)* **202**, 197.

Rubin, R. P. (1970a) *J. Physiol. (London)* **206**, 181.

Rubin, R. P. (1970b). *Pharmacol. Rev.* **22**, 389.

Rubin, R. P., Feinstein, M. B., Jaanus, S. D., and Paimre, M. (1967). *J. Pharmacol. Exp. Ther.* **155**, 463.

Rushton, M. A. (1933). *Dent. Rec.* **53**, 170.

Saeki, K. (1964). *Jap. J. Pharmacol.* **14**, 375.

Sakai, T., Cruess, R. L., and Irda, K. (1969). *Proc. Soc. Exp. Biol. Med.* **132**, 100.

Sallis, J. D., and Holdsworth, E. S. (1962). *Amer. J. Physiol.* **203**, 297.

Salvesen, H. A. (1923). *Acta Med. Scand., Suppl.* **6**, p. 5.

Samachson, J., Scheck, J., and Spencer, H. (1966). *Amer. J. Clin. Nutr.* **18**, 449.

Samiy, A. H., Hirsch, P. F., Ramsay, A. G., Giordano, C., and Merrill, J. P. (1960). *Endocrinology* **67**, 266.

Samiy, A. H., Hirsch, P. F., and Ramsay, A. G. (1965). *Amer. J. Physiol.* **208**, 73.

Samli, M. H., and Geschwind, I. I. (1968). *Endocrinology* **82**, 225.

Sammon, P. J., Stacey, R. E., and Bronner, F. (1969). *Biochem. Med.* **3**, 252.

Sammon, P. J., Stacey, R. E., and Bronner, F. (1970). *Amer. J. Physiol.* **218**, 479.

Sampson, H. W., Matthews, J. L., Martin, J. H., and Kunin, A. S. (1970). *Calcif. Tissue Res.* **5**, 305.

Sands, H., and Kessler, R. H. (1971). *Proc. Soc. Exp. Biol. Med.* **137**, 1267.

Savchuck, W. B., and Burstone, M. S. (1958). *J. Dent. Rest.* **37**, 1164.

Saville, P. D., and Smith, P. M. (1966). *Anat. Rec.* **156**, 455.

Schachter, D., and Rosen, S. M. (1959). *Amer. J. Physiol.* **196**, 357.

Schachter, D., Dowdle, E. B., and Schenker, H. (1960a). *Amer. J. Physiol.* **198**, 263.

Schachter, D., Dowdle, E. B., and Schenker, H. (1960b). *Amer. J. Physiol.* **198**, 275.

Schachter, D., Kimberg, D. V., and Schenker, H. (1961). *Amer. J. Physiol.* **200**, 1263.

Schaefer, K. E., Hasson, M., and Niemoller, H. (1961). *Proc. Soc. Exp. Biol. Med.* **107**, 355.

Schajowicsz, F., and Cabrini, R. L. (1958). *Science* **127**, 1447.

Scharf, F., Eschler, J., and Jürgens, G. (1969). *Arch. Oral Biol.* **14**, 1305.

Schedl, H. P., Osbaldiston, G. W., and Mills, I. H. (1968). *Amer. J. Physiol.* **214**, 814.

Schenk, R. K., Spiro, D., and Wiener, J. (1967). *J. Cell Biol.* **34**, 275.

Schjeide, O. A., and Urist, M. R. (1956). *Science* **124**, 1242.

Schjeide, O. A., and Urist, M. R. (1959). *Exp. Cell Res.* **17**, 84.

Schlueter, R. J., and Veis, A. (1964). *Biochemistry* **3**, 1657.

Schmidt, M. C., Lewis, A. M., Bird, E. D., and Thomas, W. C. (1966). *Amer. J. Pathol.* **48**, 439.

Schneider, F. H., Smith, A. D., and Winkler, H. (1967). *Brit. J. Pharmacol. Chemother.* **31**, 94.

Schneider, H., and Steenbock, H. (1939). *J. Biol. Chem.* **128**, 159.

Schofield, F. A., Williams, D. E., Morrell, E., McDonald, B. B., Brown, E., and MacLeod, F. L. (1956). *J. Nutr.* **59**, 561.

Schour, I. (1936a). *J. Amer. Dent. Ass.* **23**, 1946.

Schour, I. (1936b). *Anat. Rec.* **65**, 177.

Schour, I., and Rogoff, J. M. (1936). *Amer. J. Physiol.* **115**, 334.

Schour, I., and Smith, M. C. (1934). *Ariz. Agr. Exp. Sta. Tech. Bull.* **52**, 69.

Schour, I., and van Dyke, H. B. (1932). *Amer. J. Anat.* **50**, 397.

Schour, I., Hoffman, M. M., and Smith, M. C. (1941). *Amer. J. Pathol.* **17**, 529.

Schwartz, E., Panariello, V. A., and Saeli, J. (1965). *J. Clin. Invest.* **44**, 1547.

Schwartz, M., Kashiwa, H. K., Jacobson, A., and Rehm, W. (1967). *Amer. J. Physiol.* **212**, 241.

Scott, B. L. (1967). *J. Cell Biol.* **35**, 115.

Scott, B. L., and Pease, D. C. (1956). *Anat. Rec.* **126**, 465.

Scoular, F. J., Pace, J. K., and Davis, A. N. (1957). *J. Nutr.* **62**, 489.

Seidel, J. C., and Gergely, J. (1963). *Biochem. Biophys. Res. Commun.* **13**, 343.

Selinger, Z., Naim, E., and Lasser, M. (1970). *Biochim. Biophys. Acta* **203**, 326.

Seltzer, S., Bender, I. B., and Ziontz, M. (1963). *Oral Surg., Oral Med. Oral Pathol.* **16**, 846.

Selwyn, M. J., Dawson, A. P., and Dunnett, S. J. (1970). *FEBS Lett.* **10**, 1.

Seyer, J. M., and Glimcher, M. J. (1971). *Biochim. Biophys. Acta* **236**, 279.

Shah, B. G., and Draper, H. H. (1966). *Amer. J. Physiol.* **211**, 963.

Shah, B. G., Krishnarao, G. V. V., and Draper, H. H. (1967). *J. Nutr.* **92**, 30.

Shapiro, I., and Greenspan, J. S. (1969). *Calcif. Tissue Res.* **3**, 100.

Shapiro, I., Wuthier, R. E., and Irving, J. T. (1966). *Arch. Oral Biol.* **11**, 501.

Sharney, L., Wasserman, L. R., Gevirtz, N. R., Schwartz, L., and Tendler, D. (1965). *J. Mt. Sinai Hosp., New York* **32**, 201.

Shenolikar, I. S. (1970). *Amer. J. Clin. Nutr.* **23**, 63.

Sherman, H. C., and Booher, L. E. (1931). *J. Biol. Chem.* **93**, 93.

Sherman, H. C., and MacLeod, F. L. (1925). *J. Biol. Chem.* **64**, 429.

Sherman, H. C., and Pappenheimer, A. M. (1921). *Proc. Soc. Exp. Biol. Med.* **18**, 193.

Sherman, H. C., and Quinn, E. J. (1926). *J. Biol. Chem.* **67**, 667.

Sherwood, L. M., Mayer, G. P., Ramberg, C. F., Jr. Kronfeld, D. S., Aurbach, G. D., and Potts, J. T., Jr., (1968). *Endocrinology* **69**, 1074.

Shimizu, M., Glimcher, M. J., Travis, D., and Goldhaber, P. (1969). *Proc. Soc. Exp. Biol. Med.* **130**, 1175.

Ship, X. I., and Michelsen, O. (1964). *J. Dent. Res.* **43**, 1144.

Shipley, P. G., Kramer, B., and Howland, J. (1926). *Biochem. J.* **10**, 379.

Shirley, R. L., Jeter, M. A., Feaster, J. P., McCall, J. T., Outler, J. C., and Davis, G. K. (1954). *J. Nutr.* **54**, 59.

Shohl, A. T., and Wolbach, S. B. (1936). *J. Nutr.* **11**, 275.

Shohl, A. T., Brown, H. B., Chapman, E. E., Rose, C. S., and Saurwein, E. M. (1933). *J. Nutr.* **6**, 27.

Shukers, C. F., Macy, I. G., Donelson, E., Nims, B., and Hunscher, H. A. (1931). *J. Nutr.* **4**, 399.

Siegel, B. V., Smith, M. J., and Gerstl, B. (1957). *AMA Arch. Pathol.* **63**, 562.

Siekevitz, P., and Potter, V. R. (1955). *J. Biol. Chem.* **215**, 221.

Siffert, R. S. (1951). *J. Exp. Med.* **93**, 415.

Silberberg, R., and Levy, B. M. (1948). *Proc. Soc. Exp. Biol. Med.* **67**, 259.

Simkiss, K. (1961). *Nature (London)* **190**, 1217.

Simmons, D. J. (1966). *Proc. Soc. Exp. Biol. Med.* **121**, 1165.

Simpson, D. R. (1965). *Science* **147**, 501.

Simpson, F. O. (1965). *Am. J. Anat.* **117**, 1.

Simpson, F. O., and Oertelis, S. J. (1961). *Nature (London)* **189**, 758.

Simpson, M. E., Marx, W., Becks, H., and Evans, H. M. (1944). *Endocrinology* **35**, 309.

Singer, L., and Armstrong, W. D. (1959). *Arch. Biochem. Biophys.* **80**, 410.

Singer, L., Maqsood, M., Medlen, A. B., and Comar, C. L. (1957). *Arch. Biochem. Biophys.* **66**, 404.

Sisca, R. F., and Provenza, D. V. (1972). *Calcif. Tissue Res.* **9**, 1.

Slater, J. E. (1961). *Brit. J. Nutr.* **15**, 83.

Slavkin, H. C., Tetreault, C. E., and Bavetta, L. A. (1968). *J. Dent. Res.* **47**, 272.

Sledge, C. B., and Dingle, J. T. (1965). *Nature (London)* **205**, 140.

Smith, D. S. (1966). *Progr. Biophys. Mol. Biol.* **16**, 107.

Smith, R. H. (1962). *Biochem. J.* **83**, 151.

Smith, R. W., and Frame, B. (1965). *N. Eng J. Med.* **273**, 73.

Snoswell, A. M. (1966). *Biochemistry* **5**, 1660.

Sobel, A. E., and Burger, M. (1954). *Proc. Soc. Exp. Biol. Med.* **87**, 7.

Sobel, A. E., and Hanok, A. (1948). *J. Biol. Chem.* **176**, 1103.

Sobel, A. E., and Hanok, A. (1958). *J. Dent. Res.* **37**, 631.

Sobel, A. E., Rochenmacher, M., and Kramer, B. (1945). *J. Biol. Chem.* **159**, 159.

Sobel, A. E., Shaw, J. H., Hanok, A., and Nobel, S. (1960). *J. Dent. Res.* **39**, 462.

Sognnaes, R. F., and Shaw, J. H. (1952). *J. Amer. Dent. Ass.* **44**, 489.

Sognnaes, R. F., Shaw, J. H., and Bogoroch, R. (1955). *Amer. J. Physiol.* **180**, 408.

Solomons, C. C., and Irving, J. T. (1958). *Biochem. J.* **68**, 499.

Sottocasa, G., Sandri, G., Tanfili, E., de Bernard, B., Gazotti, P., Vasington, F. D., and Carofoli, E. (1972). *Biochem. Biophys. Res. Commun.* **47**, 808.

Speckman, T. W., and Norris, W. P. (1957). *Science* **126**, 753.

Spencer, H., Menczel, J., and Lewin, I. (1964). *Clin. Orthop. Related Res.* **35**, 202.
Spencer, H., Menczel, J., Lewin, I., and Samachson, J. (1965). *J. Nutr.* **86**, 125.
Spencer, H., Lewin, I., Samachson, J., and Laszlo, J. (1966). *Amer. J. Med.* **40**, 27.
Spray, C. M., and Widdowson, E. M. (1950). *Brit. J. Nutr.* **4**, 332.
Sreter, F. A. (1969). *Arch. Biochem. Biophys.* **134**, 25.
Starkey, W. E. (1971). *Arch. Oral Biol.* **16**, 479.
Steendijk, R. (1961). *Arch. Dis. Childhood* **36**, 321.
Steggerda, F. R., and Mitchell, H. H. (1941). *J. Nutr.* **21**, 577.
Steggerda, F. R., and Mitchell, H. H. (1946). *J. Nutr.* **31**, 407.
Steggerda, F. R., and Mitchell, H. H. (1951). *J. Nutr.* **45**, 201.
Stern, B., Mechanic, G. L., Glimcher, M. J., and Goldhaber, P. (1963). *Biochem. Biophys. Res. Commun.* **13**, 137.
Stewart, R. J. C., and Platt, B. S. (1961). *Proc. Nutr. Soc.* **20**, xlvi.
Stoerk, H. C., and Carnes, W. H. (1945). *J. Nutr.* **29**, 43.
Stohs, S. J., and DeLuca, H. F. (1967). *J. Ultrastruct. Res.* **6**, 3338.
Stohs, S. J., Zull, J. E., and DeLuca, H. F. (1967). *Biochemistry* **6**, 1304.
Storey, E. (1958). *J. Bone Joint Surg., Brit. Vol.* **40**, 103.
Stralfors, A. (1964). *J. Dent. Res.* **43**, 1137.
Strandh, H. J. (1960). *Exp. Cell Res.* **21**, 406.
Strates, B. S., Firschein, H. E., and Urist, M. R. (1971). *Biochim. Biophys. Acta* **244**, 121.
Suda, T., DeLuca, H. F., Schnoes, H. K., and Blunt, J. W. (1969). *Biochemistry* **8**, 3515.
Suda, T., DeLuca, H. F., Schnoes, H. K., Ponchon, G., Tanaka, Y., and Holick, M. F. (1970a). *Biochemistry* **9**, 2917.
Suda, T., DeLuca, H. F., Schnoes, H. K., Tanaka, Y., and Holick, M. F. (1970b). *Biochemistry* **9**, 4776.
Suga, S., and Gustafson, G. (1963). *Arch. Oral Biol. Suppl.* p. 223.
Suki, W. N., Schwettman, R. S., Rector, F. C., and Seldin, D. W. (1968). *Amer. J. Physiol.* **215**, 71.
Susi, F. R., Goldhaber, P., and Jennings, J. M. (1966). *Amer. J. Physiol.* **211**, 959.
Sutherland, E. W., and Rall, T. W. (1958). *J. Biol. Chem.* **232**, 1077.
Sutton, A., Shepherd, H., Harrison, G. E., and Barltrop, D. (1971). *Nature (London)* **230**, 396.
Suzuki, H. K., and Prosser, R. L. (1968). *Proc. Soc. Exp. Biol. Med.* **127**, 4.
Symonds, H. W., and Treacher, R. J. (1967). *J. Physiol. (London)* **193**, 619.
Symonds, H. W., and Treacher, R. J. (1968). *J. Physiol. (London)* **198**, 193.
Szent-Györgyi, A. (1951). "Chemistry of Muscular Contraction," 2nd rev. ed. Academic Press, New York.
Takeuchi, A., and Takeuchi, H. (1960). *J. Physiol. (London)* **154**, 52.
Takuma, S. (1960a). *J. Dent. Res.* **39**, 964.
Takuma, S. (1960b). *J. Dent. Res.* **39**, 973.
Takuma, S. (1962). *J. Dent. Res.* **41**, 883.
Talmage, R. V., Nevenschwander, J., and Kraintz, L. (1965). *Endocrinology* **16**, 103.
Taugner, G., and Hasselback. W. (1966). *Naunyn Schmiedebergs Arch. Pharmakol. Exp. Pathol.* **255**, 266.

Taylor, A. N., and Wasserman, R. H. (1967). *Arch. Biochem. Biophys.* **119**, 536.

Taylor, A. N., and Wasserman, R. H. (1970). *J. Histochem. Cytochem.* **18**, 107.

Ten Cate, A. R., Melcher, A. H., Purdy, G., and Wagner, D. (1970). *Anat. Rec.* **168**, 491.

Termine, J. D., Pullman, I., and Posner, A. S. (1967a). *Arch. Biochem. Biophys.* **122**, 318.

Termine, J. D., Wuthier, R. E., and Posner, A. S. (1967b). *Proc. Soc. Exp. Biol. Med.* **125**, 4.

Theiler, A., and Green, H. H. (1931–1932). *Nutr. Abstr. Rev.* **1**, 359.

Thomas, L., McCluskey, R. T., Potter, J. L., and Weismann, G. (1960). *J. Exp. Med.* **111**, 705.

Thomas, W. C., and Tomita, A. (1967). *Amer. J. Pathol.* **51**, 621.

Thompson, D. D., and Hiatt, H. H. (1957). *J. Clin. Invest.* **36**, 566.

Thompson, V. W., and DeLuca, H. F. (1964). *J. Biol. Chem.* **239**, 984.

Thornton, P. A. (1968a). *Proc. Soc. Exp. Biol. Med.* **127**, 1096.

Thornton, P. A. (1968b). *J. Nutr.* **95**, 388.

Thornton, P. A. (1970). *J. Nutr.* **100**, 1197.

Todhunter, E. N., and Brewer, W. (1940). *Amer. J. Physiol.* **130**, 310.

Toft, R. J., and Talmage, R. V. (1960). *Proc. Soc. Exp. Biol. Med.* **103**, 611.

Tomlin, D. H., Henry, K. M., and Kon, S. K. (1955). *Brit. J. Nutr.* **9**, 144.

Tonna, E. A., and Cronkite, E. P. (1961). *Proc. Soc. Exp. Biol. Med.* **107**, 719.

Toto, P. D., and Magon, J. J. (1966). *J. Dent. Res.* **45**, 225.

Toverud, G. (1923–1924). *J. Biol. Chem.* **58**, 583.

Toverud, S. U. (1964). *Acta Physiol. Scand.* **62**, 391.

Triffitt, J. T., Terepka, A. R., and Neuman, W. F. (1968). *Calcif. Tissue Res.* **2**, 165.

Trotter, M., and Peterson, R. R. (1955). *Anat. Rec.* **123**, 341.

Trotter, M., Broman, G. E., and Peterson, R. R. (1960). *J. Bone Joint Surg., Amer. Vol.* **42**, 50.

Trueta, J. (1963). *J. Bone Joint Surg., Brit. Vol.* **45**, 402.

Trummel, C. L., Raisz, L. G., Blunt, J. W., and DeLuca, H. F. (1969). *Science* **163**, 1450.

Tulpole, P. G., and Patwardhan, V. N. (1954). *Biochem. J.* **58**, 61.

Turner, W. A., and Hartman, A. M. (1928–1929). *J. Nutr.* **1**, 445.

Twardock, A. R., and Austin, M. K. (1970). *Amer. J. Physiol.* **219**, 540.

Twardock, A. R., Prinz, W. H., and Comar, C. L. (1960). *Arch. Biochem. Biophys.* **89**, 309.

Underwood, E., Fisch, S., and Hodge, H. C. (1951). *Amer. J. Physiol.* **166**, 387.

Urban, E., and Schedl, H. P. (1970). *Amer. J. Physiol.* **219**, 944.

Urist, M. R. (1964). *J. Bone Joint Surg., Amer. Vol.* **46**, 889.

Urist, M. R. (1967). *Amer. Zool.* **7**, 883.

Urist, M. R., and Schjeide, A. O. (1961). *J. Gen. Physiol.* **44**, 743.

Urist, M. R., Budy, A. M., and McLean, F. C. (1948). *Proc. Soc. Exp. Biol. Med.* **68**, 324.

Urist, M. R., Deutsch, N. M., Pomerantz, G., and McLean, F. C. (1960). *Amer. J. Physiol.* **199**, 851.

Vaes, G. (1968a). *Nature (London)* **219**, 939.

Vaes, G. (1968b). *J. Cell Biol.* **39**, 676.

Vale, W., Burgus, R., and Guillemin, R. (1967). *Experientia* **23**, 853.

Vanderkooi, J. M., and Martonosi, A. (1971a). *Arch. Biochem. Biophys.* **144**, 87.

Vanderkooi, J. M., and Martonosi, A. (1971b). *Arch. Biochem. Biophys.* **144**, 99.

Vasington, F. D., and Murphy, J. V. (1961). *Fed. Proc., Fed. Amer. Soc. Exp. Biol.* **20**, 146.

Vasington, F. D., and Murphy, J. V. (1962). *J. Biol. Chem.* **237**, 2670.

Veis, A., and Schlueter, R. J. (1964). *Biochemistry* **3**, 1670.

Vellar, O. D. (1968). *Scand. J. Clin. Lab. Ivest.* **21**, 157.

Vellar, O. D. (1970). *Amer. J. Clin. Nutr.* **23**, 1272.

Vincent, J., Haumont, S., and Roels, J. (1965). *J. Cell Biol.* **24**, 31.

Vinther-Paulsen, N. (1953). *Geriatrics* **8**, 76.

Volker, J. F., and Sognnaes, R. F. (1940). *J. Dent. Res.* **19**, 292.

von Hevesy, G. (1948). "Radioactive Indicators," pp. 103–106. Wiley (Interscience), New York.

von Hevesy, G., and Armstrong, W. D. (1940). *J. Dent. Res.* **19**, 318.

von Hevesy, G., Holst, J. J., and Krogh, A. (1937). *Dans. Vidensk. Selsk., Biol. Med.* **13**, 13.

Wachman, A., and Bernstein, D. S. (1968). *Lancet* **1**, 958.

Wade, P. A. (1929). *Amer. J. Med. Sci.* **177**, 790.

Walker, A. R. P., Fox, F. W., and Irving, J. T. (1948). *Biochem. J.* **42**, 452.

Walker, D. G. (1961). *Bull. Johns Hopkins Hosp.* **108**, 80.

Walker, D. G., Lapière, C. M., and Gross, J. (1964). *Biochem. Biophys. Res. Commun.* **15**, 397.

Walling, M. W., and Rothman, S. S. (1969). *Amer. J. Physiol.* **217**, 1144.

Walling, M. W., and Rothman, S. S. (1970). *J. Biol. Chem.* **245**, 5007.

Walser, M. (1960). *J. Clin. Invest.* **39**, 501.

Walser, M. (1961a). *Amer. J. Physiol.* **200**, 1099.

Walser, M. (1961b). *Amer. J. Physiol.* **201**, 769.

Walser, M. (1961c). *J. Clin. Invest.* **40**, 723.

Walser, M. (1969). *In* "Mineral Metabolism" (C. L. Comar and F. Bronner, eds.), Vol. 3, p. 236. Academic Press, New York.

Wanner, R. L., Moor, J. R., Bronner, F., Pearson, N. S., and Harris, R. S. (1956). *Fed. Proc., Fed. Amer. Soc. Exp. Biol.* **15**, 575.

Warnock, G. M., and Duckworth, J. (1944). *Biochem. J.* **38**, 220.

Wasserman, R. H. (1962). *J. Nutr.* **77**, 69.

Wasserman, R. H. (1970). *Biochim. Biophys. Acta* **203**, 176.

Wasserman, R. H., and Comar, C. L. (1959). *Proc. Soc. Exp. Biol. Med.* **101**, 314.

Wasserman, R. H., and Kallfelz, F. A. (1962). *Amer. J. Physiol.* **203**, 221.

Wasserman, R. H., and Lengemann, F. W. (1960). *J. Nutr.* **70**, 377.

Wasserman, R. H., and Taylor, A. M. (1966). *Science* **152**, 791.

Wasserman, R. H., and Taylor, A. N. (1968). *J. Biol. Chem.* **243**, 3987.

Wasserman, R. H., and Taylor, A. N. (1969). *In* "Mineral Metabolism" (C. L. Comar and F. Bronner, eds.), Vol. 3, p. 321. Academic Press, New York.

Wasserman, R. H., and Taylor, A. N. (1971). *Proc. Soc. Exp. Biol. Med.* **136**, 25.

Wasserman, R. H., Comar, C. L., and Nold, M. M. (1956). *J. Nutr.* **59**, 371.

Wasserman, R. H., Comar, C. L., Schooley, J. C., and Lengemann, F. W. (1957a). *J. Nutr.* **62**, 367.

Wasserman, R. H., Comar, C. L., Nold, M. M., and Lengemann, F. W. (1957b). *Amer. J. Physiol.* **189**, 91.

Wasserman, R. H., Taylor, A. N., and Kallfelz, F. A. (1966). *Amer. J. Physiol.* **211**, 419.

Watanabe, S. (1955). *Arch. Biochem. Biophys.* **54**, 559.

Watson, M. L. (1960). *J. Biophys. Biochem. Cytol.* **7**, 489.

Weatherill, J. A., and Weidmann, S. M. (1963). *Biochem. J.* **89**, 265.

Weber, A. (1959). *J. Biol. Chem.* **234**, 2764.

Weber, A. (1971a). *J. Gen. Physiol.* **57**, 50.

Weber, A. (1971b). *J. Gen. Physiol.* **57**, 64.

Weber, A., and Herz, R. (1963). *J. Biol. Chem.* **238**, 599.

Weber, A., and Herz, R. (1964). *In* "Biochemistry of Muscle Contraction" (J. Gergely, ed.), p. 222. Little, Brown, Boston, Massachusetts.

Weber, A., Herz, R., and Reiss, I. (1963). *J. Gen. Physiol.* **46**, 679.

Weber, A., Herz, R., and Reiss, I. (1966). *Biochem. Z.* **345**, 329.

Webling, D. D'A., and Holdsworth, E. S. (1965). *Biochem. J.* **97**, 408.

Webling, D. D'A., and Holdsworth, E. S. (1966). *Biochem. J.* **100**, 652.

Weinmann, J. P., and Sicher, H. (1955). "Bone and Bones." Mosby, St. Louis, Missouri,

Weinmann, J. P. Wessinger, G. D., and Reed, G. (1941). *J. Dent. Res.* **20**, 244.

Wells, H., and Lloyd, W. (1967). *Endocrinology* **81**, 139.

Wells, H., and Lloyd, W. (1969). *Endocrinology* **84**, 861.

Wells, H. G. (1914). "Chemical Pathology," 2nd ed. p. 402. Saunders, Philadelphia, Pennsylvania.

Wenner, C. E. (1966). *J. Biol. Chem.* **241**, 2810.

Wensel, R. H., Rich, C., Brown, A. C., and Volwiler, W. (1969). *J. Clin. Invest.* **48**, 1768.

Wergedal, J. E. (1970). *Proc. Soc. Exp. Biol. Med.* **134**, 244.

Wergedal, J. E., and Baylink, D. J. (1969). *J. Histochem. Cytochem.* **17**, 799.

Wesson, L. G., and Lauler, D. P. (1959). *Proc. Soc. Exp. Biol. Med.* **101**, 235.

Westmoreland, N., and Hoekstra, W. G. (1969). *J. Nutr.* **98**, 83.

Whitcher, L. B., Booher, L. E., and Sherman, H. C. (1936). *J. Biol. Chem.* **115**, 679.

Whittemore, C. T., and Thompson, A. (1969). *Proc. Nutr. Soc.* **28**, 16A.

Widdowson, E. M. (1962). *Voeding* **23**, 62.

Widdowson, E. M., and Dickerson, J. W. T. (1964). *In* "Mineral Metabolism" (C. L. Comar and F. Bronner, eds.), Vol. 2, Part 2A, p. 59. Academic Press, New York.

Widdowson, E. M., and Spray, C. M. (1951). *Arch. Dis. Childhood* **26**, 205.

Widdowson, E. M., McCance, R. A., and Spray, C. M. (1951). *Clin. Sci.* **10**, 113.

Widdowson, E. M., McCance, R. A., Harrison, G. E., and Sutton, A. (1963). *Lancet* **2**, 1250.

Wilde, W. S., Cowie, D. B., and Flexner, L. B. (1946). *Amer. J. Physiol.* **147**, 360.

Williams, D. E., Mason, R. L., and McDonald, B. B. (1964). *J. Nutr.* **84**, 373.

Williams, G. A., Bowser, E. N., Henderson, W. J., and Uzgeris, V. (1962). *Proc. Soc. Exp. Biol. Med.* **110**, 889.

Williams, G. A., Henderson, W. J., and Bowser, E. M. (1964). *Proc. Soc. Exp. Biol. Med.* **116**, 651.

Williams, M. L., Rose, C. S., Morrow, G., Sloan, S. E., and Barness, L. A. (1970). *Amer. J. Clin. Nutr.* **23**, 1322.

Williamson, B. J., and Freeman, S. (1957). *Amer. J. Physiol.* **191**, 384.

Wilson, P. W., Lawson, D. E. M., and Kodicek, E. (1967). *Biochem. J.* **103**, 165.

Winand, L. (1961). *Ann. Phys. (Paris)* [13] **6**, 941.

Winter, M., Morava, E., Simon, G., and Sós, J. (1970). *J. Endocrinol.* **47**, 65.

Wislocki, G. B., and Sognnaes, R. F. (1950). *Amer. J. Anat.* **87**, 239.

Wolbach, R. A. (1970). *Amer. J. Physiol.* **219**, 886.

Wolbach, S. B. (1946). *Proc. Inst. Med. Chicago* **16**, 118.

Wolbach, S. B., and Howe, P. R. (1925). *J. Exp. Med.* **42**, 753.

Wolbach, S. B., and Howe, P. R. (1926). *Arch. Pathol.* **1**, 1.

Wolf, A. V., and Ball, S. M. (1949). *Amer. J. Physiol.* **158**, 205.

Wöltgens, J. H. M., Bonting, S. L., and Bijvoet, O. L. M. (1970). *Calif. Tissue. Res.* **5**, 333.

Woodhead, J. S., O'Riordan, J. L. H., Keutmann, H. T., Stoltz, M. L., Dawson, B. F., Niall, H. D., Robinson, C. J., and Potts, J. T., Jr. (1971). *Biochemistry* **10**, 2787.

Woodin, A. M., and Wieneke, A. A. (1963). *Biochem. J.* **87**, 487.

Woodin, A. M., and Wieneke, A. A. (1964). *Biochem. J.* **90**, 498.

Woodin, A. M., and Wieneke, A. A. (1968). *Nature (London)* **220**, 283.

Woodin, A. M., and Wieneke, A. A. (1970). *In* "Calcium and Cellular Function" (A. W. Cuthbert, ed.), p. 183. St. Martin's Press, New York.

Woods, J. F., and Nichols, G. (1963). *Science* **142**, 386.

Woods, K. R., and Armstrong, W. D. (1956). *Proc. Soc. Exp. Biol. Med.* **91**, 255.

Worker, N. A., and Migicovsky, B. B. (1961a). *J. Nutr.* **74**, 490.

Worker, N. A., and Migicovsky, B. B. (1961b). *J. Nutr.* **75**, 222.

Wuthier, R. E. (1968). *J. Lipid Res.* **9**, 68.

Wuthier, R. E., Grøn, P., and Irving, J. T. (1964). *Biochem. J.* **92**, 205.

Wuthier, R. E., Cotmore, J. M., and Maron, S. S. (1968). *Calcif. Tissue. Res.* **1**, 288.

Wynn, W., Haldi, J., Bentley, K. D., and Law, M. L. (1956). *J. Nutr.* **58**, 325.

Yaeger, J. A., and Kraucunas, E. (1969). *Anat. Rec.* **164**, 1.

Yamomoto, T., and Tonomura, Y. (1967). *J. Biochem. (Tokyo)* **62**, 558.

Yamomoto, T., and Tonomura, Y. (1968). *J. Biochem. (Tokyo)* **64**, 137.

Yates, E. F. (1971). *In* "Biomedical Engineering" (J. H. U. Brown, J. E. Jacobs, and L. Stark, eds.), Chapter 1. Davis, Philadelphia, Pennsylvania.

Young, R. W. (1962). *J. Cell Biol.* **14**, 357.

Young, R. W., and Greulich, R. C. (1963). *Arch. Oral Biol.* **8**, 509.

Young, V. R., Lofgreen, G. P., and Luick, J. R. (1966). *Brit. J. Nutr.* **20**, 795.

Zambotti, V., Cescon, I., Bonferroni, B., and Bolognani, L. (1962). *Experientia* **18**, 318.

Zamoscianyk, H., and Veis, A. (1966). *Fed. Proc., Fed. Amer. Soc. Exp. Biol.* **25**, No. 2, 409.

Ziskin, D. E., and Applebaum, E. (1940). *J. Dent. Res.* **19**, 304.

Zull, J. E., Czarnowska-Misztal, E., and DeLuca, H. F. (1965). *Science* **149**, 182.

SUBJECT INDEX